PRAISE FOR
BABY GOT BACK IN HER PANTS

Baby Got Back In Her Pants delivers a well rounded and inspirational message. It's truly a motivational dynamo! Step into the pages of this book, let the kind and caring support from Christin Bummer fuel you to take action, and you will most definitely be impressed with what you can achieve.
~John Pierre
Author of *The Pillars of Health* and *Strong, Savvy, Safe.*
Co-founder of LivingWithHarmony.org

Christin Bummer has gifted us with her unique system for implementing an enjoyable plant-based diet. She offers **an action plan that turns daunting into flaunting**.
~ Dr. Michael Greger
New York Times Best Selling Author of *How Not To Die* and *How Not To Diet*

I have found **Christin Bummer's passion, energy and willingness to help** others reclaim their health inspirational not only to me but everyone she meets and shares her story with. In *Baby Got Back in Her Pants*, you'll find the easy path to health improvement. When you are done reading you will say **"I can get healthier just like Christin did!"** The journey to health is not just about saying no to certain foods but **recognizing stress, overcoming food cravings and so much more.** It is all there for you in *Baby Got Back in Her Pants*.
~Paul Chatlin
Founder of PBNSG, Plant Based Nutrition Support Group

This is **not just a weight loss program** focusing on what to eat (although that's crucial!) but the hows and the whys too. The array of tools are phenomenal! I'm a month in and my jeans are looser and my acid reflux is GONE!
~Tina P.

I love the book! **I really like the workbook-style aspect.** It definitely helps to go deeper and make real changes.
~Kate P.

I love how all the information is so positive and personal. We all want to be healthy, happy and get the most out of life. **This book is the first time ever that I found the information I needed** to not only get me on the path, but keep me going through some challenging situations.

I had already been vegan and just began eating whole food plant based, but had so many questions. There was a lot of information on the internet but I needed more than recipes.

Baby Got Back In Her Pants addresses so much more than the food, I always knew it had to be more than the food. Living your life with joy, eating healthy and delicious food, holding yourself accountable, moving to get the happy hormones flowing, truly being grateful for all you have around you, this book truly inspired me to live my best life.
~Rise A.

Today is Day 50. I'm down 16.2 pounds **without any restriction on food portions**. My clothes are getting loose and I can honestly say that **I've had no cravings whatsoever! A miracle!** I have been trying to get on track for at least 5 years with no success at all!
~Karen M.

Baby Got Back In Her Pants really guides you through steps to prepare you for success, starting from scratch. If you're struggling to **find motivation that lasts**, this book has the answer. The success stories are inspiring, and there's **super clear information** about what foods to eat. Finally, the book guides you with what to do when perfection rears its ugly head and you've had a slip, which has been so helpful as **an all-or-nothing approach spells trouble for me.**
~Jody C.

It's like **your best girlfriend coaching you along**, and helping you, and rooting for you! It means the world to see someone that went through it who's helping pull you along
~Donna V.

Baby Got Back In Her Pants delivers a **clear, concise guide to healthy eating,** and a balanced lifestyle of **compassion and acceptance without judgement.** This book will inspire and motivate you to adopt a clean, plant-based lifestyle that will enhance your life in multi-faceted ways.

And it's simple and fun!!! Get off the roller coaster and live your best life right here and right now (in your favorite pants). You won't regret it!
~ Jeni F.

Baby Got BACK IN HER PANTS

Disclaimer

This book contains the ideas and opinions of its author. It is intended to provide helpful general information to help the reader make informed decisions. It is not intended as a substitute for any treatment that may have been prescribed by a doctor. If the reader needs personal medical, health, dietary, exercise, or other assistance or advice, the reader should consult a competent physician and/or other qualified health care professionals. The author and publisher specifically disclaim all responsibility for injury, damage, or loss that the reader may incur as a direct or indirect result of following any directions or suggestions given in the book.

Mention of specific companies, organizations, or authorities in this book does not imply endorsement by the author or publisher, nor does mention of specific companies, organizations, or authorities imply that they endorse this book, its author, or the publisher.

Published by The Nourishing Life, LLC

Copyright © 2020 by Christin Bummer

All rights reserved. No part of this book may be reproduced or used in any manner without written permission of the copyright owner except for the use of quotations in a book review. For more information, address: chris@theForeverDiet.org.

First American Edition November 2020
9 8 7 6 5 4 3 2 1

Foreword by Michael Greger, M.D., FACLM
Edited by Tracy Jenkins
Designed by Heidi Caperton

Color Paperback ISBN 978-1-7359602-1-0
Black and White Paperback ISBN 978-1-7359602-2-7
eBook ISBN 978-1-7359602-0-3

Library of Congress Control Number: 2020921876

www.theforeverdiet.org

Baby Got Back in Her Pants

A Simple Plan
to Thrive on a Plant-Based Diet

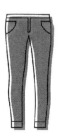

CHRISTIN BUMMER

"Never doubt that a small group of thoughtful, committed, citizens can change the world. Indeed it is the only thing that ever has."

~MARGARET MEAD

Dedication

For Mike, who meets and exceeds my enthusiasm
for even my wildest dreams.

For Carolyn, who reminds me every day about the
precious gift of living in this very moment.

For Dad, who taught me that all things are possible.

For Mom, who taught me to always leave
a place better than I found it.

For Heather, who inspires me to live
boldly and to always say YES!

Special Acknowledgements

To **TammieBeth Montgomery**, without whom this book would not exist. You believed in my message, guided me through uncharted territory, and breathed life into this book. You have generously shared your talent, expertise, and professionalism to create a truly effective and influential work of art. I am forever thankful.

To **Karen Casalone**, without whom my journey would have been so very different. You have been my constant cheerleader, devoted confidant, and an integral part of my journey as a coach and as a business leader. You have championed me and challenged me while gently reminding me of the importance of patience and self-care. I am truly fortunate to have you in my life.

With Gratitude

It takes a village to create a movement, and I owe a debt of gratitude to those who have come before me and to those who have influenced my journey every step of the way. You've proven that real change is possible. You've proven that people always deserve better and that they are willing to take action to create change. There are so many great people in this world, and you are just a few of my very favorite people. You stepped in at just the right time, and I am so thankful for your message and support.

T. Colin Campbell, Ph.D. who taught me that I don't need to eat animals to survive.

Caldwell Esselstyn, M.D. who taught me that my family history would not be my fate.

John Pierre (aka J.P.) who taught me the infinite power of love and compassion for all.

Michael Greger, M.D. who provided a resource (NutritionFacts.org) to answer all of the questions I had when I began my journey.

Stacey Martino who taught me how to truly love and appreciate everyone in their own place on their own journey.

Russell Brunson who provided me a megaphone to reach the masses.

Mandy Morris who taught me that healing is the foundation for health, and to heal the world, all we need is love.

My editor, **Tracy Jenkins**, whose insight, inspiration, and gentle guidance made *Baby Got Back In Her Pants* a better book.

Barbara Rolls for your groundbreaking research on calorie density in *Volumetrics*.

Dr. Alan Goldhamer and **Dr. Doug Lisle** for your profound insight and roadmap to freedom inside *The Pleasure Trap*.

CLAIM YOUR FREE WORKBOOK

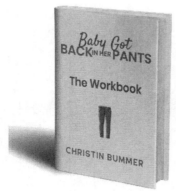

Don't wait another minute! Use this workbook to record your thoughts and plans so that you can get into action right away!

AND A FREE AUDIOBOOK

No more excuses!
As a free gift for purchasing the book, you can take your motivation to go! Listen wherever it's convenient.

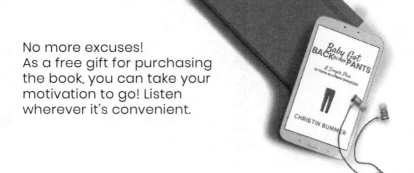

www.theforeverdiet.org/book-bonuses

Table of Contents

Foreword xi

Introduction xv

Chapter 1. Bye Bye 20s, Hello Hypertension. 1

Chapter 2. Creating Massive Motivation. 13

Chapter 3. One Small Thing 31

Chapter 4. Fill Her Up, High Octane Please! 47

Chapter 5. Green Means GO!. 65

Chapter 6. Kicking Cravings to the Curb 83

Chapter 7. If Only Pasta Grew on Trees 101

Chapter 8. Making Your Life
Interesting with P.L.A.N.T.S. 111

Chapter 9. A for Activity 129

Chapter 10. It Takes a Village. 139

Recipes 149

The Path Forward. 181

About Christin. 185

Quick Favor. 187

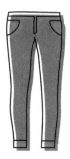

FOREWORD

The best kept secret of medicine is that the body heals itself if we create the right conditions. And when we stop doing things that created sickness in the first place.

~ DR. MICHAEL GREGER

At age 65, my beloved grandma, Frances Greger, was diagnosed with end-stage heart disease. She had already had so many bypass operations that the surgeons had essentially run out of plumbing, and the scarring from each open-heart surgery had made the next one more difficult. When they finally ran out of options, they sent her home to wait out her remaining days. Soon after she was discharged, she caught a segment on *60 Minutes* about the work of Nathan Pritikin, one of lifestyle medicine's early pioneers who had been gaining a reputation for reversing terminal heart disease and had just opened a new center—a live-in program where everyone was placed on a plant-based diet and then started on a graded exercise regimen.

What happened next is chronicled in Pritikin's biography: She managed to make the trek, arriving in a wheelchair, to be one of his first patients. Within three weeks, she wasn't just out of her wheelchair, but she was walking ten miles a day on her own. Thanks to a healthy diet and lifestyle, she was able to enjoy another 31 years on this planet with her six grandkids, including me. The woman who had once been told by doctors she only had weeks to live didn't die until she was 96 years old. Her near-miraculous recovery not only inspired one of those grandkids to pursue a career in medicine but granted her enough healthy years to see him graduate from medical school.

By the time I became a doctor, giants like Dean Ornish, M.D., president and founder of the nonprofit Preventive Medicine Research Institute, had already proven beyond a shadow of a doubt what Pritikin had shown to be true.

Using the latest high-tech advances—cardiac PET scans, quantitative coronary arteriography, and radionuclide ventriculography—Dr. Ornish and his colleagues showed that the lowest-tech approach—diet and lifestyle—can undeniably reverse heart disease, our leading killer.

Dr. Ornish and his colleagues' studies were published in some of the most prestigious medical journals in the world. Yet medical practice hardly changed. Why? Why were doctors still prescribing drugs and using Roto-Rooter-type procedures to just treat the symptoms of heart disease and to try to forestall what they chose to believe was the inevitable—an early death?

The question that haunted me during training was this: *If the cure to our number-one killer could get lost down the rabbit hole, what else might be buried in the medical literature?* I made it my life's mission to find out and that's what pushed me to found NutritionFacts.org.

We have tremendous power over our health destiny and longevity, and given the right conditions, our bodies have an incredible power to heal. What we eat is the number one determinant of how long we live. What we eat is what determines most whether we'll die prematurely. What we eat is what determines most whether we become disabled or not.

When we fuel ourselves with a whole food plant-based diet rich in a wide variety of vegetables, fruits, legumes, whole grains, nuts, and seeds, we have the potential to prevent and even reverse a host of our most common diseases: heart disease, diabetes, kidney disease, and more. But, sometimes, just having that information may not be enough, and people can benefit from a guide to help them embrace long-lasting diet and lifestyle changes. I say long-lasting because there's no point in making drastic changes only to fall back off the bandwagon and end up worse off than when you had started. Thankfully, the single best way of eating for weight loss may just so happen to be the safest, cheapest way to eat for the longest, healthiest life.

Christin Bummer has gifted us with her unique system for implementing an enjoyable plant-based diet and she offers an action plan that turns daunting into flaunting. *Baby Got Back in Her Pants* pairs Christin's wealth of information with an accessible, workbook-style format that readers will find motivating and supportive.

My grandmother's transformation was the reason I went into medicine—to do for other families what Pritikin did for mine—and I'm thrilled to see Christin doing the same, using her own journey to continue inspiring others.

There are no gimmicks, no quick-fix solutions, no diet supplements. Christin reminds readers of the simple power to heal themselves using healthy, whole, plant foods.

It's not what you eat today or tomorrow that matters, but what you eat over the next several months and years, so you have to find lifestyle changes that fit into your lifestyle, and Christin can help you do just that.

To your great health,

MICHAEL GREGER, M.D., FACLM

Founder of NutritionFacts.org and *New York Times* bestselling author of *How Not to Die* and *How Not to Diet*

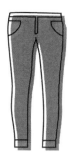

INTRODUCTION:

Are You Done Being Stuck?

> *Perfectionism is a twenty-ton shield that we lug around thinking it will protect us when in fact it's the thing that's really preventing us from taking flight.*
> ~ BRENE BROWN

I am so happy that you're on this journey with me! We're about to have a whole lot of fun! This will be different from everything you've tried in the past, and you're going to be thrilled you said YES! The world of lifestyle change can be daunting and it doesn't have to be. I will help you understand exactly what to do and how to get started.

I have designed this book to be a condensed version of the most important information you need to embrace a plant-based lifestyle and to experience its benefits to the max. The changes I made to my food in 2011 were daunting at first. I struggled a bit, but I adapted quickly. The changes I saw in my life as a result were nothing short of miraculous! It is my greatest wish for you to experience even a taste of what I've accomplished, be inspired by the success stories of my clients, and enjoy your very own transformation.

I'll be offering some guidelines and suggestions for you to follow to see the results that are waiting for you (if you choose to accept them). Are these suggestions in the form of hard and fast rules? No. Are they rules that will get you kicked out of the club if you don't follow them? No! If I've learned anything in the past 9 years on my whole food plant-based lifestyle journey, it's that the pursuit of perfectionism is a fast-track to failure. It's time to let that idealism go right out the window!

I'm not your boss and I'll never try to shove you into a box. Think of me as your mentor and your coach and your new BFF! I won't offer a demanding set of rules, but I will offer guidance, share experiences, and I will cheer you on along your journey. I will show you reliable systems that work, and I'll explain why so it finally makes sense to you!! That being said, *you* are the one who makes the final call. No one can be pushed, guilted, or shamed into success. Guilt and shame have no place here whatsoever. They'll just keep you stuck.

My approach is to offer you a map to take the most fun and smooth adventure possible with the least amount of detours we can manage.

Before we get into exactly what I suggest, it'll be easier for you to understand just one more thing: Why I do what I do. There are a million things I could do with the 24 hours I get every day. And yet here I am, spending my time writing to you, my new friend. There's a big reason, and once you understand this reason, everything I teach you is going to make a whole lot more sense.

My father-in-law was a meat 'n potatoes Pittsburgher, born and bred. He had Iron City beer flowing in his veins, and he was the life of the party. Every guy in town considered him his best friend. He was full of chivalry and kindness. He'd do anything for anyone, and that went triple for his family.

> To the world you may be one person, but to one person you are the world.
>
> ~ *Bill Wilson*

There's nothing he talked about more than wanting grandchildren. My husband and I weren't planning to have kids, and he had a really hard time letting go of the hope that we'd change our minds. He'd tease all the time about what a great mom I was to our dogs, and imagine how great I'd be with a baby.

When my husband and I cleaned up our diets in 2011, he commended us and also made it very clear that he wanted no part of it for himself. He saw us ogling fresh tomatoes and homegrown asparagus, and he was grossed out. He saw us turn down hot dogs on the 4th of July and the cake at my cousin's wedding, and he was puzzled. He also saw us slim down and become more active, more enthusiastic, and more energetic than ever before. He witnessed how we both came alive. And yet, he made it clear this was a spectator sport when it came to him.

He had only one rule when it came to food - "*If it's green, I don't eat it.*" And he was a man of his word!

The only vegetable he ever ate was corn.

He'd had a big beer belly for as long as I'd known him. He went through two knee replacements to regain mobility. He watched friends succumb to heart disease, diabetes, and cancer over the years, many of them way before their time.

We gently shared stories of survival, of reversing disease, of overcoming cancer, and of becoming heart attack proof. Still, he saw no need to modify his diet or lifestyle, even as he neared 70.

When he saw my husband and me get lean and fit, he'd say, "*That's great for you guys. I'm sure it's the healthiest way to be, there's no doubt in my mind. But I could never do it.*"

And so he didn't.

He had served time in the Navy after trade school, and

he worked his whole career in the VA hospital. He saved for retirement and was looking forward to building his dream home with his wife and enjoying their golden years together.

He had 2 granddaughters who put the sparkle in his eye, and he was over the moon when we announced that ours was on the way. He used to pat my growing belly all the time, somehow already having a special connection with that baby before she was even born.

His eyes welled up with happy tears when he held her for the first time and we announced she was to be named after his little sister who had died in childhood. If he'd had a daughter, she would have been named the same, but having two boys instead never gave him the chance.

He held her only a few more times after that. When she was 6 weeks old, he was diagnosed with pancreatic cancer. We had a head-spinning, world-churning experience, and only 6 more weeks after the initial diagnosis, my baby girl was waving good-bye to him in a coffin.

Yes, I am aware that technically babies that young can't actually wave, but I saw it with my own eyes. She was only three months old. She looked over the edge of her ErgoBaby carrier that kept her close to me. She looked at him in the coffin. She smiled and she waved. And I lost it.

There's not a day that goes by that I don't think about what he used to say, "*I'd rather die than eat healthy.*"

Did he *really* mean that?

Did he know the choice he was making?

Would he have chosen differently if he did?

Did he really choose pizza and beer over quality time

with me? His wife? His sons? With his newborn granddaughter?

If he knew how amazing she is today, and how much fun she is to be around, would he have figured out a way to eat a few more salads?

What if I could have gotten through to him?

I'll never know the answer to those questions. And I've learned to be ok with that.

You see, I wasn't a coach back then. I didn't know what I know now. I didn't know how to meet him where he was, and to help him make tiny changes that could have impacted his longevity.

And while I'll never know if I could have "saved" him, he drives me and motivates me to this day. You see, no matter who I'm working with, I see my client as a grandmother with grandbabies who need her to rock them to sleep. I see a mom with kids who need a strong role model. I see a sister who has nieces and nephews looking up to her.

I see a powerful woman trapped inside a prison of shame and blame. I see a girl with walls up all around her because she's been hurt too many times or because people haven't seen her for the amazing person she truly is.

I see people for who they truly are. And I know that I can help them.

I do what I do with such passion because I know that *there are people in your life who need you.* They want you around for as long as possible, and they want you to feel young and lively and full of energy. There's no greater gift you can give your loved ones.

I know that I can and do make a difference in the lives

that I touch, and you deserve the chance to live the life that is waiting for you. It's never too late.

So when you say to me, "*I'd rather die than eat one more vegetable*," or "*It's so hard to eat healthy when everyone else is not*," you'll never see me roll my eyes.

You'll never hear me argue with you.

You'll never see me give up on you.

I know you just haven't yet seen things the way that I see them. And that's ok. I know when the chocolate cake calls your name, you're not evaluating it against how many good years you want to spend with your loved ones. No one actually thinks like that.

But I'll show you how to retrain your brain to work for you, not against you. You'll be faced with temptations from now until the end of time, and you will want a toolbox to help you navigate those situations.

So when you express challenges, when you "fess up" to slip-ups or to going off-plan, you'll never hear me scold you. You'll see me standing *with* you, every step of the way, meeting you wherever you are, guiding you if you'll let me. I'll be helping you become the version of you that you deserve to be.

My mission is to help you live the fullest life that you possibly can, but that's not all. It's not just for your benefit. I care about you more than you know. But the truth is, I do what I do because I care about your kids and your grandkids, even if they haven't been born yet. I do what I do because every kid deserves to grow up with parents and grandparents who are an active part of her life.

Every person alive today has more ability to impact their health and longevity than they realize. And you, my friend, while special in your own ways, are no exception to this rule.

The diets that you've tried in the past haven't served you, have they?

If I had to guess, there were a few crucial elements missing: fun, sustainability, tools for real motivation, and perhaps accountability. If any one of these elements is missing, you're doomed to failure. So if that's what you've experienced in the past, don't sweat it. You're not alone. You're in good company, and you needn't struggle anymore.

Diets might have started you on your path, and maybe you've seen some success with weight loss. But were you restricting your food or trying to fight against your body's natural tendencies, preferences, and desires? Were you trading one symptom at the expense of another? Short term weight loss at the expense of heart health or diabetes, for example?

There's no need to trade one problem for another, and we're not going to fight those natural tendencies anymore, okay? It's time to do things differently.

> There's something you need to know right up front. This program is not just about food. I repeat - this is not just a diet.

There's something you need to know right up front. This program is not just about food. I repeat - this is *not* just a diet. I hate to break it to you, but having my recipes, checklists, and menus are no guarantee of success in any way.

The food is important, and I promise to teach you everything you need to know about eating whole food plant-based (starting with what that even means and how many people get it wrong)! But it's not just about knowing what to eat. It's about learning how to make it *fun*, practical, and *sustainable* so that you can enjoy doing it. When you can approach it from that angle, you can actually keep it up for the long term!

You see, it's just like having a GPS device. You can put in your destination, but until you actually start moving, you won't get any useful directions! It's only once you're in motion that you start to see whether you're on the right path or not. As long as you're in motion, you'll get continual feedback as to whether you're staying on the right path. Use this feedback for what it is - information - and just keep going.

In the past, people have asked me for the *Cliffs Notes* version of TransformU, my online training program. They wanted only the most important, big concepts that will really move the needle so they could get started right away. They've asked me, "*Where exactly do I even start adopting or refining a plant-based lifestyle?*" The answer is in your hands right now.

This book will help you find your motivation again. It will help you get into the right headspace. It will hand you the tools to make this easy, which in turn, will make it sustainable. Lifestyle really is a practice, and there's no such thing as being "done" with it. So the more you can embrace this idea from the beginning, the more success you're likely to see. It will take more than 24 hours to turn your ship around, so give yourself a little grace and a little patience so that you can actually put these ideas into practice. If you pace yourself, you should be able to get through the content in the next 30 days, having plenty of time to implement the tools as you go along.

If you could use a little more support as you work your way through this book, and beyond, I have some fabulous options for you!

One is my Facebook Community which you can access at www.facebook.com/groups/BabyGotBackInHerPants. Join us to meet real people who are on this journey with you. Get some ideas for meal prep and recipes, and find support for navigating the real world as you take the next step in your journey. Ask questions when you hit a rough patch, and enjoy the cheers of your peers as you celebrate your accomplishments!

Another great way to get support is to join my online coaching programs. You'll find helpful suggestions for food preparation and menu planning as well as ongoing coaching, motivation, and accountability.

To learn about the options, visit:

www.theforeverdiet. org.

I don't want to waste any time getting you to your results, so I've taken hours and hours of education and boiled them down to only the most important stuff you need to take action. I know you'll want to read this cover to cover, but the most successful plan is to work through the content a little bit at a time and give yourself som time in between chapters to do the assignments and to let things sink in.

So dive in, digest the material, print out the downloads, and most importantly - take action! Any action will do. I should let you know right up front that this is not a spectator sport. Don't let this become a "shelf help" book that you just start reading and then let it collect dust while you go about your days frustrated with your weight.

Can we be done doing that, please?!

This is your life. You are the star of the show and it's time for you to take the stage! I have designed a companion workbook so that you can speed up your progress by taking an active role. You can download the workbook and other bonuses from my website at www.theforeverdiet.org/book-bonuses. You'll see action steps at the end of each chapter. Use those to take action. Grab a pen or pencil, answer the questions right in the book or in your workbook, and take an active part in this process to get the most out of it.

My goal is to help you to get into those pants that are way too snug right now. You know, the ones you used to squeeze into on a good day, but now you can't even button them up? Those are the ones we've got in our sights.

My question to you is, *"Are you done being stuck?"*

Let's make a pact here and now, shall we?

> Raise your right hand and repeat after me.
>
> I, _____, *am done dieting.*
> *I am done feeling guilty.*
> *I am done beating myself up.*
> *I am done trying to seek a quick fix.*
> *I am done treating my body like a garbage disposal.*
> *I am ready to treat my body with respect.*
> *I am ready to seek food that makes me feel good in the short term and the long term.*
> *I know that food is medicine.*
> *I know that I can do this.*
> *I want to do this.*
> *I will do this.*
> *I am strong.*
> *I will not give up.*
> *I will keep going until I achieve my goals.*

Nice job. You're off to a great start already.

The device is on. The destination is set. You've got the roadmap in your hands. We're ready for action.

HEY, PANTS, WE'RE COMING FOR YOU!

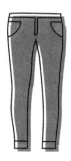

CHAPTER 1

Bye Bye 20s, Hello Hypertension

Mirror Mirror on the wall,
I'll always get up after I fall.
And whether I run or walk or crawl,
I'll set my goals and achieve them all.

~ UNKNOWN

I grew up a happy, healthy kid. I was always active and fairly athletic. I started gymnastics at age 2, excelled at swimming, fell in love with volleyball in junior high, and rode horses competitively at Cornell University. I prided myself on my muscular body, yet I longed to be slimmer than I was.

After college, my activity level dropped dramatically, but it wasn't until I was in my late 20s when the weight started to creep up. Little by little my muscle was transforming to flab, and I didn't like it. I tried everything to get a handle on it including dieting, extreme exercising, and every reasonable suggestion I learned along the way. I saw temporary improvements many times over, but nothing lasted.

By my early 30s I was getting pretty frustrated. I didn't see a doctor regularly because I was married to one and quite frankly, I didn't see the need. If I had gotten sick, I'd pop into an urgent care facility, get my prescription, and go about my day. I noticed after a few of these visits in recent years that my blood pressure was going up each time. Not drastically, but it was ticking up bit by bit, undeniably. No one seemed to notice. No one was worried about it, but I knew enough to be concerned.

My family has a terrible history of heart disease, high blood pressure, high cholesterol, and type 2 diabetes. There I was at 32, wondering if I was heading down that path too.

I wanted a solution, but I had no idea where to look. I was already doing the things I knew to do - eat lean meat, low-fat dairy, not too many carbs, and lots and lots of exercise. And yet it wasn't working. It didn't add up.

My friend introduced me to a book she'd read that was all about the link between dairy and cancer. She couldn't recall many details to explain further, but I was totally intrigued. I was shocked to hear those two things in the same sentence: dairy and cancer. I couldn't wait to get the book in my hands. It was called *The China Study* by T. Colin Campbell. I read the book cover to cover in a week's time. The book explains decades of research which suggest that it's not necessarily the animal fat that's the most problematic for cancer, but the animal protein.

Wait. What?

I thought animal protein was good! I was eating a ton of it, trying to stay healthy.

By the end of the book, I'd given up meat and dairy. I knew that was part of the definition of veganism. I didn't even know what the rest of it meant at the time, but I was all in.

It was only a few days later when someone else recommended the book *Prevent and Reverse Heart Disease* by Caldwell Esselstyn, M.D.

Come again?

Reverse heart disease?

You mean it's not a one-way diagnosis?

I was floored!

I'd always thought cancer, diabetes, and heart disease were just things some (older) people got, and lucky people didn't get. I knew eating deep-fried Twinkies would fast-track your path there, but I had no idea you could actually prevent or reliably reverse it.

Those two books set me off on a journey that changed

my life forever. I changed my diet over the course of one week (while on vacation in Alaska, no less). When I got home I scheduled a physical to get some baseline bloodwork.

I tend to make careful decisions. I wanted all of the numbers to evaluate the changes I was making. On the day of my check-up, I walked down the hall to the exam room, and as I approached the scale, the dread rose to my ears.

It had been at least 5 years since my last visit. I took off my shoes and my socks, and would've taken off my jewelry and my scrunchie if the nurse had given me time to do it! Instead, I sucked in my gut and held my breath.

I stepped on the scale and the number was higher than I'd been accustomed to. A lot higher. When I put on the paper "gown", the disgust really surfaced.

There is no flattering way to sit on a medical table in a napkin. The whole picture was just depressing. My boobs were sagging without my cute underwire bra, my belly had a new roll I hadn't noticed before, and for the first time, I desperately wished I was wearing Spanx.

Just as I was getting pretty sick of looking at myself, wondering where the hell my body had gone, the doc came in. After the small talk, he asked me what I'd been up to. He asked about my activity levels. I could tell he was tiptoeing around something. And then it came out - I was heavier than I'd ever been. UGH!

I was *shocked* at that. My weight had crept up to my highest weight ever, and that wasn't even the concerning part.

When he said my blood pressure was 140/90, I was *totally surprised*! I knew it was rising, but it had never been that high. Ever. He checked it 3 times before I would even accept the reading. He handed me a script for blood pressure pills, and my jaw hit the floor.

> My weight had crept up to my highest weight ever, but that wasn't the concerning part

My mom was on blood pressure pills. My dad had been on blood pressure pills since he was 19. But me? I never really had anything wrong with me!

My grandfathers had both died of heart disease, my grandmother had suffered from Alzheimer's, and I knew high blood pressure was even more predictive of a heart attack than high cholesterol.

Crap.

My family history was dead ahead, waiting for me with open arms. There was nothing but a platter of grandma's chocolate chip cookies to comfort me.

My doctor wasn't supportive of my plant-based solution, but that made me dig in my heels even more, to prove him wrong. He gave me 6 months to give it a try. He made it very clear if I came back in 6 months with the same blood pressure, I'd have no choice but to begin taking medication.

I walked out of that office determined to try to do things

the natural way. I didn't want that diagnosis, I did not want to be dependent on drugs for survival at such a young age. I was determined to escape it. But I had no idea if it would really work for me.

I had already been eating healthier for a couple of weeks by then, but this took it to a whole new level. Could I really give up cheese and ice cream forever? I didn't know if I could. I didn't know if I even wanted to. Would it be worth the sacrifice?

I pulled my too-tight pants back on and marched out of that office knowing that somehow, whatever it took, I at least had to try.

I wasn't ready to accept the diagnosis, so instead I accepted the challenge and went all-in. I decided to do my very best for 30 days and then reevaluate.

I was nervous and excited all at the same time, but I knew if I didn't at least attempt this experiment, I'd always regret it.

I went home and started treating my body like a finely-tuned machine I wanted to last a lifetime. I didn't want it to fall apart. I didn't want to run out of gas and be stranded on the side of the road watching the rest of my life go by while I was held back by disease and limitations.

I started eating more salads. I started drinking more water. I started filling up on veggies and sweet potatoes and quinoa. I even tried kale for the first time and after a few failed attempts, it wasn't half bad!

I got rid of the animal products that were clogging my arteries. I let go of the cheese I never thought I could let go of. I walked away from dairy ice cream for a temporary experiment. Nine years later (at the time of this first printing), I'm still carrying out the experiment. The results are looking good as they come in.

While it happened quite quickly for me, the change was a bit overwhelming at first. One morning I was eating eggs and bacon for breakfast and the next it was oatmeal every day for a month until I figured out some more interesting options. It was only a couple of weeks before my first family event - a 4th of July BBQ, and I was freaking out. I'd never been to a family picnic without eating burgers and hot dogs, and I really wasn't sure how it was going to go.

My husband and I picked up some veggie burgers at the grocery store along with a couple of Lara Bars in case of an emergency. I was thrilled to find that I could also eat the watermelon, corn on the cob, and raw veggies and I certainly did not go hungry. In fact, I didn't feel like I was missing out at all.

I was relieved that we were able to field the questions with a few basic explanations. Back in my early days, I was what you'd call a "vegangelist", someone who tries to convert everyone they come across to veganism. I felt so enlightened, so empowered, and I was flabbergasted that this life-changing information was not on the six o'clock news! I wanted everyone to know what I'd come to know, and it was my deepest wish for my friends and family to come on board the health train with me!

Of course, it didn't exactly work that way. Let's just say it made for some awkward family picnics. I ran up against some skepticism, judgment, and opposition. Over time, I learned to appreciate that everyone is on their own journey. It is not my job to change anyone who doesn't wish to change. And yet I've been able to make it my job to facilitate anyone who wants desperately to change!

It's always heart-wrenching to see those I care the most about choosing to dig a deeper hole toward disease and disability, and it's also the most rewarding thing in the world to work with someone when they first become awake, when they start to realize the power they hold. It brings me so much joy to see people come alive and to engage with life in a way they never have before!

Bye Bye 20s, Hello Hypertension

CLIENT SPOTLIGHT
MEET AMY

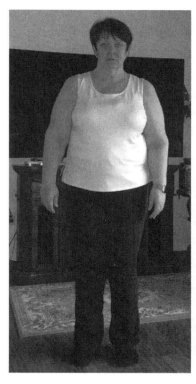
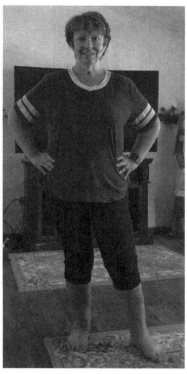

For the first two years of adopting a plant-based diet I tried following Dr. Fuhrman, then Engine2, then Dr. McDougall, and others. You name it, I tried to do it. I was bouncing from book to book trying to absorb it all but nothing was sticking. I was just digging a deeper hole and getting frustrated. I even tried a few other plant-based programs, and just didn't find a fit. I often felt self-conscious and judged and would retreat back into my shell.

I endured abuse as a child and sadly, I felt like it was my fault. I felt judged and punished. I was later raped at knifepoint, and I kept it a secret because I was afraid of being judged. I lived in shame, and I hid.

So when I came across judgment in a Facebook group, I high-tailed it out of there. It just wasn't for me. I could see a little success from time to time, but I was trying so hard to be perfect that eventually I would hit the drive-thru and start gaining again.

Just when I thought things were hard enough, I lost my uncle who I was very close to, and it sent me reeling. I gained a lot of weight again, and I felt so defeated. It was almost torturous because I had a lot of knowledge. I knew what to do, but I just couldn't help myself.

And then I found Christin Bummer! I fell in love with the videos in her program, and everything made so much sense. It's explained and organized so well that I was able to actually do it this time, and I could sustain it! In hindsight, I didn't need to read a bunch of different books to get all of the information. She's done the work already and put it all together in one place. It's super- condensed and easy to understand!

I finally embraced the idea that each bite is either helpful or hurtful, and just focusing on one meal at a time has kept me going for the first time. I stopped striving to be perfect, and here I am eating cleaner than I ever have.

It wasn't just the food, but I found a whole new approach to my life completely. I really resonated with Christin's lessons on positivity and I've gained a new perspective on life in the process. I've learned to look at the past, and instead of reliving the trauma, I'm able to see how far I've come, and how much this lifestyle has helped me to heal in so many ways.

I've stayed away from the scale, so I don't know how much weight I've lost so far, but I can see my clothes getting baggier all the time! And the best part is, when I went back to my doctor for my check-up, my numbers were better than ever. In just a few months of following this program, I reversed my hypertension and I dropped my cholesterol by 40 points. I'm just so excited to finally feel like I can do this!

I found a lot of success thanks to the support of the Facebook community and I bet you will too! Will you join me? Say hello so I know who you are and let us know how we can help you.

~AMY

READY, SET, ACTION!

One of the biggest things that helped Amy was to tap in to a community where she found positivity and support. When you're surrounded by love and compassion, your chances of success skyrocket!

Your first assignment is to join my Facebook community: The Plant-Based Success Club where you will find a judgment-free zone full of other like-minded folks who are taking back control of their health and happiness.

Your tasks:
1. Join my Facebook community: www.Facebook.com/groups/BabyGotBackInHerPants
2. Introduce yourself.
3. Ask questions.
4. Get ideas, and share support for others!

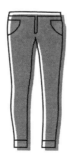

CHAPTER 2:

Creating Massive Motivation

*What great thing would you attempt
if you knew you could not fail?*
~ ROBERT H. SCHULLER

This plant-based lifestyle has so much potential to really and truly change the way that you experience the rest of your life! This is a big deal! It's powerful, and if you're reading this book, you already know that. You may have already dabbled with a plant-based diet, or maybe you've been working on some version of a plant-based diet for a long time but for some reason, just haven't been able to stick to it for the long haul. In any case, I'm going to suggest that for one reason or another you picked up this book because you haven't been able to reach all of your goals yet.

> You already know what happens when you get pulled off track. Now it's time to see what happens when you stay motivated and you keep going until you realize your dreams

Before we even start talking about the food, we've got to dive into an essential piece - how to tap into some powerful motivation so we can overcome this wiring and continue working toward our goals effectively.

Come with me as we create some massive motivation that's very specific and personal to you. When you're done with this chapter, you will have drawn out your most powerful driving factors. You'll have a concrete tool to call upon this motivator at any time. Doing the work in this chapter will help keep you on track, always moving toward your goals instead of giving up when the going gets tough.

You already know what happens when you get pulled off track. Now it's time to see what happens when you stay motivated and you keep going until you realize your dreams. Are you ready?

We're trying to find the motivation that's driving you so you can keep coming back to it over and over again. We're going to uncover your why, the thing that will keep you strong when you don't feel like you can be strong anymore. That "why" is going to remind you it's worth it. You are worth it, even when it's uncomfortable or inconvenient.

I'm going to ask you a few questions, so grab a pen and actually write down these answers as we go along. I know I don't normally tell you what to do, but this time I mean it - go grab go grab your workbook and a fresh pen! Download the workbook at www.theforeverdiet.org/book-bonuses or write right along in this book, whichever you prefer. Even if you already know your why, you'll want to do this exercise. You may be surprised by the results.

I'll offer a series of questions for you to work through sequentially. Once you read the question, take your time and write down your answer. Write the first thing that comes to mind. This does not have to be a long essay. You can even make bulleted phrases or thoughts, and you can come back to it later and expand upon it. Just be sure to start it. Don't skip this section. It's too important!

Okay, are you ready?

What would you do if I handed you ten million dollars right now?

Think about it for a moment - I just handed you ten million dollars. No strings attached. How are you going to spend it? There's no right or wrong, don't censor yourself - just roll with it. Go!

_____

_____

_____

_____

_____

See, the thing is, most of us wake up every morning, go to a job, work in our own businesses, or do something to make money without any real thought as to what the bigger purpose is.

Sure, you need money to pay your bills, but did you realize all of your bills are choices, too? What kind of house are you paying for? Are you working like crazy so you can live in a nice home that's a little outside of your comfortable budget? Or do you live in a more modest home and drive a high-end vehicle?

_____

_____

What do you prioritize when it comes to entertainment? Do you have plenty of money to travel or do you spend your money elsewhere?

_____

_____

_____

Creating Massive Motivation

What do you do with your spare time?

_____

_____

_____

Do you give generously to your favorite causes, or do you always feel bad when they look for donations and you say, "I wish I could, I just can't right now"?

_____

_____

_____

Be a little more specific now. What else can you buy with ten million dollars that you aren't already buying?

_____

_____

_____

_____

_____

The choices we make are simply a reflection of our values and our driving forces. They tell us what is important to us.

What do you do differently, now that money is no longer something you worry about? I know this feels far-fetched but play along for a few minutes. If this does ever happen to you, the last thing you want to do is be unprepared! We talked about how you're going to spend your money. Now I ask, how do you spend your time?

_____

_____

_____

What is your purpose for going to work? And if you're already retired, don't think you're off the hook. In fact, you'll have even more work to do with this question! You've already put in your time. You've worked a career, you've saved for retirement. For your golden years. What is it you want to do with them? Write it down….

_____

_____

_____

_____

_____

_____

We're really getting somewhere now. Doesn't it feel different getting out of bed in the morning if you're going to work on achieving your dreams? Among the things you've written down so far, you probably have some hierarchy. Go ahead and put a star by the two most important things you've written down so far. Take a look at the dreams or aspirations that are really important to you.

Creating Massive Motivation

Some version of these things is actually your driving force, your purpose. Now, with your big purpose in mind, with those big dreams and aspirations you would carry out if money was no object...

How does your health play a role in that picture? In other words, are you limited in what you can do with your big purpose if you don't have your health?

_____

_____

_____

Now, what if instead of ten million dollars, I handed you a voucher for a lifetime of fantastic health?

What if:
We wipe away any current or future chronic diseases - type 2 diabetes, your high cholesterol, high blood pressure?
We take away your aches and pains?
We erase your family history and you now come from a long line of long-living people?
We reverse the signs of aging?
We wash away cancer?
We could eliminate the likelihood of dementia or stroke?
Your body would shrink to its ideal size?
You could be strong, capable, and independent?
You'd never worry about your weight again?

Pause and write down how you would feel if I handed you such a voucher.

_____
_____
_____
_____
_____

My friend, the ten million dollar thing was pie in the sky. I admit that. It was just part of an exercise. But, the clean bill of health? The ideal body shape and fitness level, freedom from aches and pains and chronic disease? It's achievable. I see it happen every day with my own eyes: A clean bill of health. Body image is no longer an issue. Self-esteem and self-confidence are sky-high.

This is all yours for the taking!

All right, here's where it comes together.

What do you do differently with your life knowing that health and weight are no longer a concern for you? That you have a strong, capable, and functional body?

_____
_____
_____
_____
_____

We tend to focus on things like money, career, and aspirations. And we often take for granted our health. And yet, even with all of the money in the world, we can't fulfill our dreams if we don't have our health!

We often get up every day and go about making money, uninspired because we're forgetting the big picture, our bigger purpose. One day blends into the next and we start to get bored with it all.

When it comes to our health the same exact thing happens. We set out to "get slimmer" or "get healthier" without any strong conviction about it. What's the point of reaching your ideal body weight unless you're going to do something with that capable body?

You know, when people think about goals, they think about things like losing a certain number of pounds or fitting into a certain size of clothing. Maybe they think about completing a 5K or a half marathon or hiking a special distance. I hate to break it to you, but none of those are goals. They're just items you may or may not check off your list one day. All you really have is a wish list.

I don't know about you, but it takes more than a to-do list for me to get it to-done!

I'm a bright person. I'm motivated fairly easily. I have a supportive husband and a lot of resources (a gym membership, some home gym equipment, access to healthy groceries, and a safe place to walk or jog if I choose to). Despite having plenty of tools at my disposal even in 2011, the only thing I was losing was confidence, and the only thing I was gaining was weight. This went on for years!

Until I got a scary diagnosis. The moment I saw a script

for blood pressure pills with my name on it, I changed. In a moment I shifted. It was *enough* to push me into action, and within 4-5 weeks I hit the weight loss goal that had eluded me for years. I had goals all along the way but I wasn't hitting them. I wanted to be thinner, I didn't like how I felt, I desperately wanted to change, and I sure was trying. And then all of a sudden, everything clicked.

Why?

I had tapped into massive motivation. I didn't want to go down that path. I was slamming the brakes on hard so that I could pivot and take a different path. It was not my time to head toward disability, and I wasn't going that way without a fight.

You may have already had a scary diagnosis, or maybe even a few. You may already feel like you've got tons of motivation, and you may be wondering what's wrong with you.

Nothing is wrong with you. You just don't have enough of that motivation to reach your tipping point yet. Most coaches try to coerce people into changing their eating habits by reminding them of all of the scary things that can happen if they don't change.

I am not most coaches.

When you can start to actually envision your life and all of the beauty that awaits, you can shift. When you can see yourself in your new life, doing the things you love to do, participating in the things that are important to you, you can shift. When you can see the possibility and regain the hope of becoming the very best version of yourself, you can shift. You can take action, evaluate your progress, adjust as needed, and keep going until you arrive. There is no other way.

When you can shift your perspective and start going about this with a renewed sense of purpose, with an eye on the bigger picture, then you have a greater chance of success. I am convinced this is one of the reasons so many people struggle over and over again. They *know* what to do, but they just aren't *doing* it consistently, and it's because they haven't yet locked in to the motivation that will keep them moving forward no matter what.

> They *know* what to do, but they just aren't *doing* it consistently, and it's because they haven't yet locked in to the motivation that will keep them moving forward no matter what

So now it's time for you to find yours. It's time to lock it into your sights. Go back and review your answers from the beginning of this exercise. Look past the surface. What is really important to you? What are the things you'd have or do if money and health were no object?

Summarize them here:

_____

_____

_____

These are your driving factors. You may want to lose x amount of pounds, but what you wrote above is the real reason *why* you want to do it. We're going to take it one step further and convert your why (your summary above) into an affirmation. This statement will help guide your decisions over the next month and beyond.

Some examples to get you started:

I am filling my body with health-promoting foods so I can...
I treat my body with love and respect because I am...
_____

_____

_____

Play with a few different variations until you find something that really feels authentic to you. It should feel aspirational and truthful, even if a smidge far-fetched at this moment in time. We're setting the stage for the future in every decision that we make today. This is your chance to write your own future. It's a perfect time to aim high!

I'm so proud of you for sticking with me! You won't regret going through this exercise.

Creating Massive Motivation

CLIENT SPOTLIGHT
MEET KAREN

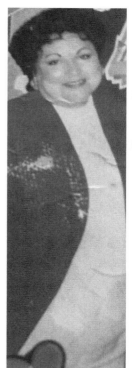
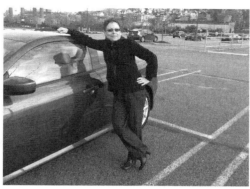
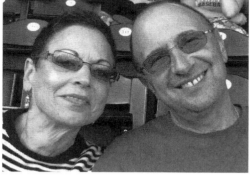

I grew up as a chubby child with a tiny petite mom who made me conscious of my weight and appearance before I even hit puberty. She was always slim, well-dressed, and proper, and I became supremely aware of the fact that I never measured up to her expectations. She labeled me a chocoholic and I never relinquished the label! I started dieting when I was in the 6th grade and I continued for the next 5 decades.

I entered the workforce and fought my way up the ladder as the first woman in a man's world in the pharmaceutical industry. Being the only woman, I felt pressure to eat like the guys ate - steak, potatoes, hard liquor. I poured my energy into my work where I found success and satisfaction, but the result was a nagging reminder that I was growing wider every year.

When my husband Jim was diagnosed with cancer at age 51 and given 2 to 3 years to live.... my whole world stopped on a dime. My priorities shifted in a moment, and I became hyper- focused on supporting his journey to healing.

I had always been teased for my bad cooking. When we first got married, I would cook dinner for Jim, and here's how most nights went: I'd take a taste of it. He would take a taste of it. And without saying anything, he would follow me to the garbage can and we'd go out to McDonald's!

I tried my best, but when my husband became ill, I had to figure it out. I couldn't keep feeding him rich and fatty restaurant meals and fast food!

I read everything I could get my hands on about optimal nutrition for cancer. It led me first to juicing, then to veganism, and eventually to a whole-food plant-based diet. I started following the 21 Day Kickstart from PCRM and Chef AJ and found success, but I was still totally focused on the food. Truth be told, I only joined Christin's programs to be supportive. But wouldn't you know, I ended up losing 15 more pounds in the first few months?!

It was because I started to understand the whole picture better, and I really embraced everything she taught. It all made so much more sense than the way I'd learned it before, and when I rewired my brain for positivity and success, the weight just melted off. I'd had a muffin-top that I thought was a permanent reminder of how big I used to be. But it's gone now, and I've maintained my weight loss more easily than ever before.

When I first walked through her exercise on Motivation, I answered each question honestly and without judgment, and I was shocked at how quickly I was able to get to the root of what was driving me. I have been able to tap into this motivation easily every day since, and I'm sure it is a huge reason for my success.

I've released a total of 100 lbs over the years. Now, when I walk in the room, people often refer to me as tiny, and I still look over my shoulder to see who they're referring to. Even after all this time, it's hard to identify with my new body but it's getting more and more real every day! The weight loss was a huge focus, and now I realize it was just a symptom and a side-effect of my day-to-day decisions.

It wasn't just the weight though. I'm a different person both inside and out. My husband and I have been through some dark and scary times together, and I suffered from clinical depression and frequent anxiety. I have continued to work on myself and improve myself from the inside out. I no longer rely on anything other than my own skills and my PLANTS targets to get me through life. I released the need for antidepressant medications. I no longer use alcohol, caffeine, or chocolate as coping crutches! This year Jim celebrates his 72nd birthday, 21 years after his diagnosis! We are both stronger, healthier, and happier than we've ever been.

This motivation exercise set me off on a path that led to losing my last 15 pounds and keeping it off for over a year and counting. So, will you at least try it? Pause here until you complete the exercise!

~KAREN

Creating Massive Motivation

READY, SET, ACTION!

Karen had been in weight loss programs for decades and plant-based programs for another 5 years before she began working with me. She had a wealth of information, but she hadn't quite reached her goals yet. She set her preconceived notions aside and remained opened to learning. She jumped in and completed the assignments. To this day, she swears this one assignment was such an eye-opener that it gave her a completely different perspective on this path, and from that day forward her decisions about how to take care of herself became infinitely easier. Are you ready for things to get a whole lot easier too?

Here's your assignment:

1. Refine your affirmation statement until you're happy with it. Write it on the following page.
2. If you'd like help refining it or putting a positive spin on it, ask for help in the Facebook group.
3. Keep this book handy, in a visible location. *Pick it up every day* and read this affirmation statement out loud to yourself every day for 30 days. Keep referring back to it even as you continue through the rest of the book.

This is the massive motivation you've been looking for. And now, my friend, it's GO TIME!!

My affirmation statement:
_____
_____
_____
_____
_____

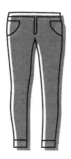

CHAPTER 3:

One Small Thing

One small thing doesn't seem like a lot
One small thing, work with the time you've got
Soon, one small thing becomes two
After two, perhaps another few
Then one small thing is not so small
One small thing can be the biggest thing of all.

~ KRISTIN CHENOWITH, RARITY
MY LITTLE PONY: THE MOVIE

When it comes to achieving your goals, one of the most important pieces is motivation. Finding your why and getting to the root of what's driving you is crucial for setting yourself up for success. What you've accomplished in the last chapter is *huge*!

Unfortunately, it's not the only thing.

Wanting something isn't enough to manifest it, is it? Thinking about a goal, wanting it, and moving toward it doesn't guarantee that it will come to fruition. While there are a lot of things we want, there are only a few things that we're willing to work for. There are even fewer things we're willing to claim for ourselves.

I've worked with many wonderful clients over the years, and I've watched them evolve and transform no matter how their journey began. No matter where or how you see yourself now, please know that there is a next level for you! There are some folks who start off all fired up and raring to go. Maybe it's because they've reached their rock bottom, they've had a scary diagnosis, or maybe they're just tired of feeling crappy and they're finally ready for help.

There are other clients who approach this lifestyle change the same way they approach stepping on a scale: with a heaping portion of doubt and terror with a side of raw resistance. They start off a bit timid and unsure. An outsider might think they're half-assing it, but there's more to it than that.

Sure, they'd like to feel better. Yes, they'd love to drop 25 lbs (or 125 lbs) and be able to shop in a regular clothing store. But here's the real problem: they doubt it will actually work. They doubt it's any different from the other hundred things they've tried. Even if they believe it can work for others, they doubt it will work *for them*.

The truth is, they carry a heavy burden wondering whether they're even capable of experiencing anything other than the life they've known so far: a life full of disappointment, of overweight, of frustration, of falling short even when they try so hard. Often there's trauma, rejection, depression, anxiety, or all of the above.

The result is a predictable snowball of doubt, more discomfort, more disappointment, and even more doubt about ever being able to pull out of it and see the results they hope to see.

One of the essential pieces to achieving success is believing that you can be successful. Sometimes the truth really is that simple.

Think of it like buying a Lottery ticket. You know the odds are slim, very very slim, and yet deep down, you still hope that you're going to win. If you didn't carry at least a small speck of belief that you could win, you'd never spend money to buy the ticket. That's a fact.

No matter what negative messages you have flying around in your head right now, I also know that there are positive messages too. There is at least a glimmer of hope, and at least a speck of belief. Do you know how I know this?

It's because this book is in your hands. If you're reading these words, it means that somewhere deep inside, you have a belief that this might actually work for you. You've decided that it's worth a try, and here you are, giving it your best shot. In my mind, you're already a winner!

Okay, since we can see there's at least a glimmer of hope, how do you go about fostering that belief so that you move closer and closer to realizing your dreams?

There are five steps in this process, and it goes like this:
1. Defining a goal that you would like to accomplish
2. Identifying all of the steps to achieving that goal
3. Ordering the steps by priority or chronologically
4. Selecting the first step to take
5. Taking the first step - the One Small Thing

You have identified your driving factors, and you have summarized them into an affirmative statement or two. Your statement may or may not feel specific enough to be actionable, which is totally fine. In this next part, we're going to turn it into a goal. Of course, you may have multiple goals, and you can use this process for each of them individually. For now, just select one goal to focus on, and work through that one from start to finish.

Let's say you've realized that you'd like to make decisions that are beneficial for your body as well as your mind and spirit. Your affirmation might be: "*I treat my mind, body, and soul with love and respect because I am setting an example for my daughter!*"

That's a fantastic affirmation! So let's see how we can massage that into a goal.

How about this? "*I will gift myself 20 minutes of self-care every day for the next 30 days.*"

Now that's starting to feel more specific and actionable, right?

Even with an understanding of what drives us, meaningful goals to shoot for, and our eyes on the prize, we can't make any progress until we get into motion. Many people get to the point of creating a goal, and then they can't quite figure out what to do about it, so they never get started.

There is a trick to getting started, and the good news is that it's easier than you might think. The key is to reduce the perceived distance between here and there. To lower the effort required to make that first step.

> The key is to reduce the perceived distance between here and there

Think back to your goal, and now break the goal down into smaller, bite-sized chunks. Keep breaking it down, spelling it out, step by step, until you can brainstorm every single step that has to happen. Ideally, most steps only take about 10-15 minutes to complete. That's how small they should be broken down.

Now go back through and identify the first five steps that need to happen sequentially, or in order of priority, and number them 1-5.

Take a look at step #1, and do that today!

In my self-care example, my goal is to do 20 minutes of self-care every day for 30 days.

To make that happen, I would come up with all of the steps that it'll take to accomplish this:
- Research meditation
- Find guided meditations
- Brainstorm ideas for self-care
- Find or create free space on my calendar for self-care
- Actually schedule some kind of self-care every day
- Consider finding a self-care accountability buddy
- Write down all the reasons I deserve self-care
- Make a self-care vision board to keep me motivated
- Set alarms on my phone so I don't forget
- Make a calendar to track daily self-care
- Set up a reward system for completing my goal for this month
- Create a consequence that will deter me from skipping out on my daily plan
- Ask my partner to help me by preventing distractions for 20 minutes each day

So then I would identify these as my first 5:
1. Brainstorm ideas for self-care
2. Write down all the reasons I deserve self-care
3. Find or create free space on my calendar for self-care
4. Actually schedule some kind of self-care every day
5. Create a consequence that will deter me from skipping out on my daily plan.

Can you see the monumental difference between saying "*I've really got to get better about my self-care*" to declaring a goal, "*I'm going to dedicate 20 minutes/day to self-care for the next 30 days*"?

Can you also see the difference between declaring that goal and taking action on it *today*?

It's so easy to procrastinate, and when the goal feels too big or too hard, we'll put it off indefinitely. We'll wait till life settles down, till work is less crazy, till this project is done and we have "more time." And yet no matter how much we convince ourselves that this is realistic, that time never actually comes!

Having a goal is good. Having a step by step plan to attack it is better. Having a plan that is broken down into bite-sized pieces is best.

When each action step only takes 5-15 minutes to complete, and it's as easy as "brainstorm ideas", now you've got something that you can take action on today. Your goal here is to make your tasks so teeny weeny that you can't *not* complete it! Is this making sense?

> I have the tasks for each room broken down into bite-sized pieces so I can tackle them in 10 minutes or less

Let's take another example from everyday life so you can see how this plays out. I use this strategy to keep my home and office organized, and to tackle major projects. If my house is a disaster, it can be daunting to clean it up.

So I have a checklist I created using the system I described above. I broke the house into rooms. Each room has a list of all of the steps required to clean it. And then I put the steps in order. So when it's time to tackle something, I never ever think about cleaning the whole house. If I did that, I'd get overwhelmed and never get started. Instead, I just pick one room, glance at the list, and do the first thing on the list. And here's the important part - I forget about the rest! Until I'm ready for the next step, it's off of my radar. This is key!

I have the tasks for each room broken down into bite-sized pieces so I can tackle them in 10 minutes or less. I even set a timer sometimes - 10 minutes to tackle one specific section of my office, or to clear out old emails, or whatever it is! If I had the task to "organize the playroom" for example, it would be so daunting I'd never even get started. But if I have 10 minutes, I can go in there and at least put all the books away. I can check it off my list and I feel great!

> If you're stuck in a rut, I would almost definitely guess it's because you've been feeling like the way out is too big a step

In my home, I often start in the kitchen. I set a timer for 10 minutes and get as much done as I can. First, I'd do all of the dirty dishes. Then, I'd clear off the counters, clear the table, dry the dishes, and then put them away. I'd tackle the miscellaneous things that land in the kitchen - like the mail, keys, school work, etc - and put it all in its place. If I'm feeling ambitious, I'll sweep and mop the floors and if there's time, I'll move on to the next room. This used to never happen all in one day for me and yet it's shocking how much I can accomplish in 10 minutes when my energy is focused and directed!

That's what it's all about for our health and wellness goals too - chunk it down so small you'd be crazy not to take action. Then take action. Then celebrate! Enjoy that little victory. That's a dopamine hit, and you've earned it!

If you're stuck in a rut, I would almost definitely guess it's because you've been feeling like the way out is too big a step. Maybe you've dug yourself such a deep hole that you can't even see the top anymore. Maybe you come up with a plan to buckle down starting Monday, but you never quite get started, or you're giving up by Tuesday because it's too hard.

The key to getting out of that rut is to reduce the height of that first step - just break down your goal into something so small and manageable that you can't help but get it right. It's about taking a logical approach, one small step at a time, to get right back on track.

This is a strategy I've nicknamed One Small Thing. Next time you find yourself somewhat stuck, I want you to think, *"What's one small thing I can do today to get closer to my goals?"*

Baby Got Back in Her Pants

CLIENT SPOTLIGHT
MEET JULIE

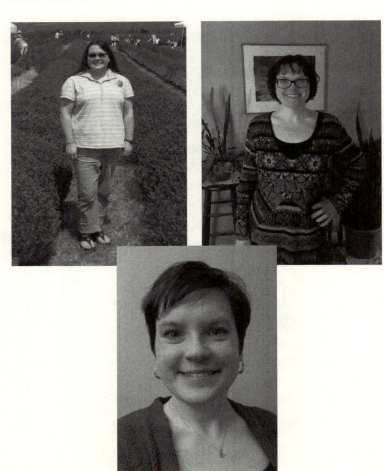

You know how a lot of people long to look like they did in high school? Well, not me. I currently weigh less and am more physically and mentally fit than I was as a teenager. My "glory days" were not so glorious. I spent my entire childhood being bullied because of my weight and I was very shy. By high school, I was obese, in a constant state of anxiety and feeling like I didn't fit in.

In the middle of that already brewing storm, at the age of 15, I was diagnosed with type 2 diabetes, still mainly known at that time as "adult-onset" diabetes. I knew that my body was not normal for a teenager. I was sent to a dietician and told to count carbs. I remember sitting across the lunch table from a classmate. I would watch her eat her fill of snack foods that I formerly enjoyed while I ate my carefully portioned, carb counted meal. And when my meal was finished, as I sat there still hungry, I'd look at my friend's thin, lean body and think, "why can't I just be normal?"

This disease followed me into adulthood despite my trying to ignore it. By my late twenties, my physical and mental health were spiraling out of control. I went to the doctor and was put on medication for my diabetes as well as for PCOS, high cholesterol, and high blood pressure. It was a punch to the gut. I thought to myself, "these meds are for old people, not someone in their twenties!" Knowing that my current path was leading to a most certain early death, I decided to change course.

Since embracing a whole food plant-based diet, I have experienced sustainable weight loss for the first time in my life. I no longer take any medication. My blood pressure, triglycerides, and total cholesterol are in the normal range. My A1C readings and fasting blood sugar readings no longer fall in the diabetic category. And while I may still have pre-diabetes, I know that I am on the right track to completely reverse my metabolic dysfunction.

I've adopted an active lifestyle, and am very proud that I have become an accomplished runner. I started out running 50 steps at a time and progressed until I was ready for my first 5K. I've since completed many 5K and 10K races as well as three 10 mile races, four half marathons, and even a full marathon.

As much as I'd like to say that this is the point where I rode off into the sunset, my story is not that simple. Even after having adopted my WFPB lifestyle, the pull toward using food to cope with the stress of life was extreme. I would be very hard on myself for even slightly straying off- plan. You see, I tend to be perfectionistic, and when I fall short of the high expectations I set for myself, I throw in the towel. Before long, I propel myself into a downward cycle of weight gain, guilt, depression, and binge eating. This happened time and time again, and I just could not understand why I wasn't able to be consistent with healthy choices. Knowing what to do wasn't enough. Something was missing.

Working with Christin has had a profound effect on my life and my outlook. I was able to let go of my perfectionism and my all-or-nothing attitude, instead focusing intensely on the One Small Thing strategy. I broke my goals down into bite-sized chunks, and I stayed in the moment so that I could tackle just that one thing that was in front of me. This greater presence and focus has resulted in tremendous success ever since. My self-esteem and confidence have improved through approaching my goals in this way. I have lost over 20 pounds, and I know that I am capable of sustaining my healthy lifestyle. Christin helped me to see that mindset and mindfulness are truly so important to achieving success.

Even though I would have told you several years ago that I had all of the information I needed, it wasn't until I fully embraced all of the Forever Diet concepts that I finally saw long term success. It's about so much more than just the food, understanding the science, or knowing what to do. It's about knowing that you have the tools to make it happen in the real world. The guidance and support of this program have made all the difference for me. I know that my healthiest and happiest days are ahead of me.

I used to fall into the trap of thinking that the teeny goals weren't worthy of working toward, or they weren't anything to get excited about. So I'd set lofty goals and put off starting them because I was overwhelmed (and full of excuses!) Once I adopted the One Small Thing strategy, I've been taking teeny steps to work toward my lofty goals, and it feels so good! Your turn!

~JULIE

READY, SET, ACTION!

Ok, so here's your assignment:

1. Think about your goals or anything you've been wanting to tackle in your life that you keep putting off.
2. Choose one goal to work through.
3. Brainstorm all of the steps to making that happen.
4. Prioritize them in order.
5. Identify One Small Thing you can do today!
6. Go do it!
7. Take a peek at the next few steps and plug them into your calendar for this week!
8. Share your plan in the Facebook group so we can hold you accountable!

My Goal:

_____
_____
_____

The steps it'll take:

-
-
-
-
-
-

-
-
-
-
-
-

The top 5:

1.
2.
3.
4.
5.

The One Small Thing I can do today is:

_____

Go do it and report in the Facebook group so we can do the happy dance with you!

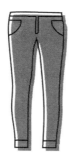

CHAPTER 4

Fill Her Up, High Octane Please!

*I already know what giving up feels like.
I want to see what happens when I don't.*

~NEILA REY

When I embraced a whole food plant-based diet for the first time in 2011, just after reading *The China Study* and *Prevent and Reverse Heart Disease*, I lost 15 pounds in about 3 weeks. This was a first for me, and I was ecstatic. For the first time ever, I didn't lose weight from burning calories, I did it by *eating* calories.

I was making the right food choices which were helping my body to heal, and it was really showing on my waistline. Without even understanding all of the details at the time, I lost weight from what I'm about to teach you right now: calorie density.

This is simply the number of calories per unit of measure of food. In other words, it's a measure of how much energy you get out of what you put in. For the sake of consistency and simplicity, we measure this in calories per pound.

All foods have a different calorie density, and we can group foods together into categories of similar calorie density in order to understand how this affects us in real life. See the chart on the next page to make this crystal clear:

The first category is vegetables, which have about 100 calories per pound. This includes vegetables like artichokes, asparagus, green beans, broccoli, zucchini, water chestnuts, peppers, tomatoes, eggplant, mushrooms, salad greens, onions, etc.

Whole fruit comes in around 300 calories per pound. There's a range of calorie densities among the various fruits, but 300 calories per pound is a good rule of thumb. This category includes apples, bananas, berries, oranges, watermelon, mango, papaya, pomegranate, and more.

Calorie Density
WEIGHT LOSS KEY

Calories Per Pound

100	VEGETABLES (NON-STARCHY)	
300	FRUIT	
400	POTATO, CORN, SQUASH, OATS	*Go*
500	WHOLE GRAINS, RICE, PASTA	
600	BEANS & LEGUMES	
750	AVOCADOS	
*2800	NUTS AND SEEDS	*Caution*
1200	ICE CREAM	
1400	BREADS, BAGELS, WRAPS	
1600	CHEESE	*Stop*
1800	SUGAR, CRACKERS	
2500	CHOCOLATE	
2800	NUT BUTTERS	
4000	ALL OILS	

Figure 1: Calorie Density Key

Did you catch that "whole" part? We'll come back to that in a little bit. It's an important distinction.

Starchy vegetables like corn, potatoes, sweet potatoes, and squash such as acorn, butternut, and kabocha average about 400 calories per pound.

Whole grains average around 500 calories per pound. When I say whole grains, I mean actual whole grains like brown rice, quinoa, millet, wild rice, black rice, amaranth, oat groats, etc. This does not refer to products or processed foods that are labeled "whole grain." That distinction trips up a lot of well-intended healthy eaters and is a source of unexplained weight gain or stubborn weight loss. It's so important that we'll cover more of that in a later chapter, I promise.

Beans and legumes come in around 600 calories per pound. Examples include beans, peas, and lentils. My favorites include black beans, chickpeas, pinto beans, and kidney beans, but there are many more to choose from. Packed with protein, these are definitely an essential part of the whole food plant-based diet.

Up until this point, everything I've mentioned: non-starchy vegetables, fruit, starchy vegetables, whole grains, and legumes, all fit into a healthy and balanced whole food plant-based diet! If you went shopping in only these sections of the calorie density chart from here on out, you would consume a diet that is rich in nutrients and low in calories. This is how you can use food to your maximum benefit by gifting your body with maximum nutrients and melting off excess weight.

Continuing down the chart, you'll see the calorie density start to climb into a zone where it becomes more problematic for overall health as well as for optimal weight. Let's skip right to ice cream at 1200 calories per pound. I realize you're not often weighing out the decision to eat a bowl of kale or a bowl of ice cream. But if you were, you'd find the ice cream is leaving you with twelve times the calorie density. Every time you choose watermelon over ice cream, you're taking in only a quarter of the calorie density.

Let's face it, we all know eating bowls of ice cream day

Fill Her Up, High Octane Please!

after day isn't going to end well. But then we have the bread, bagels, muffins, pita, and most flour products at 1400 calories per pound. I'm gonna stop right there...

Bread and bagels are more calorically dense than full-fat dairy ice cream. Did you catch that? Just checking.

Can you see where carbs start to get a bad reputation? The carbohydrates from *processed* grains are in a completely different category than the carbohydrates from *whole* grains. It's not carbohydrates that are crushing our weight loss efforts. It's the other C-word - calorie density!

Do you have the strength to continue? Don't worry - I do have good news with all of this, I promise!

Sugar and pretzels and crackers weigh in at 1800 calories per pound. Pretzels! Crackers! These are the things that you're likely to grab from the snack table thinking they're not so bad. Clearly, it's all relative, and there are worse choices, but not as many as you might think.

And then we jump to chocolate at 2500 calories per pound.

Here's a surprising one - nuts, seeds, and nut butters come in at 2800 calories per pound. Whoa, Nelly! Suddenly you'll understand why I could never lose weight when I was eating my beloved peanut butter and chocolate treats. I was packing in so many calories even in a tiny package that made it impossible to shed the pounds.

Oopsie!

Last but not least, we've got oils. All oils. Yes, even avocado oil, coconut oil, and cold-pressed extra virgin olive oil that claim to be heart healthy. Even those weigh in at 4000 calories per pound. Holy moly, that's intense! I know this probably isn't what you wanted to hear today, but I'll reassure you that it just may be the best news you've heard in a long time.

Okay, take a deep breath. Inhale... Exhale... We're getting to the good part.

This principle of calorie density and your implementation of it can catapult your success with a plant-based lifestyle. If you've struggled so far, I would venture to guess that you weren't eating according to these principles. If you're familiar with calorie density and you're still not seeing the results you'd like to see, stick with me because you're about to find some opportunities for improvement that will help you move forward.

Clearly, we don't always eat our food in pounds at a time, so the numbers may feel a little abstract until you're used to playing around with them. Let's take a look at a real-life example. Non-starchy vegetables have about 100 calories per pound whereas ice cream has around 1200 calories per pound. You might think, "*I'd never eat a pound of ice cream (in public)*!" That may be so, but did you know that a pound of ice cream is one pint which equates to about 3 cups? Let's say you could eat half of that in one sitting. Is that fair?

If you eat half a pound of ice cream, you'll take in 600 calories. If I eat a whole pound of non-starchy vegetables, which could be 12-15 spears of asparagus I'll still only get 100 calories. You get 600 calories and I get 100 calories. Big difference, right?

Put differently, I could eat a pound of vegetables, half a pound of potatoes, and a pound of fruit to equal the same

Fill Her Up, High Octane Please!

600 calories you'll get from half a pound of ice cream. That's about 3 cups of salad, 2 small to medium potatoes, and 1 ½ cups of watermelon for the same 600 calories that you get from 1 ½ cups of ice cream. Ooohhh.

See where I'm going with this? When you stick with foods that are lower in calorie density, you can eat a whole lot more of them and you'll be losing weight without watching your portions or starving yourself. Make this choice all day every day and the weight will be melting off your body faster than you can fill your belly!

> When you stick with foods that are lower in calorie density, you can eat a whole lot more of them and you'll be losing weight without watching your portions or starving yourself

Let's look at this same principle another way. Let's see what this volume of food looks like where it counts - in your body.

Figure 2, on the next page, shows you what calorie density looks like in practice. These five stomachs all contain 500 calories of food. But you can see the volume that 500 calories takes up varies wildly based on the food.

In the stomach on the far right, you've got 500 calories of fruits and vegetables. It fills up 2 liters which is about the size of an average distended stomach - ie, a happy full belly! This could be one big giant salad or it could be a generous bowl of vegetable stir fry with mango and watermelon for dessert.

Calorie Density
WHAT 500 CALORIES LOOK LIKE

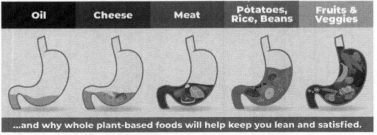

Figure 2: Calorie density in the body

In figure 2, you've got 500 calories of starch like potatoes, rice, and beans. This could be baked sweet potatoes, air fried potato wedges, or a giant pot of butternut squash soup and a bowl of rice. Any combination really fills up the stomach nicely.

Once we get past the starches, the story changes a little. In the next image, you see 500 calories of red meat, fish, and poultry. Here, the same 500 calories are keeping your stomach only half full. Since this 500 calorie meal won't even begin to initiate your stretch receptors signaling the end of the meal, you'll have to eat more food in order to feel full. In doing so, you'll consume way more calories.

And then, we get to cheese. Suddenly, 500 calories doesn't fill you up at all, does it? To *feel* full on this stuff, you'd have to eat 4-5 times that amount. You don't want to see what happens when you eat four pounds of cheese in order to feel full! Just trust me on that one.

So even if you made a conscious choice to skip the salads and eat your cheese or ice cream because you'd rather have

500 calories of deliciousness than 500 calories of something you perceive as less delicious... Even if you made that choice, there's a major flaw. You will not feel full on those 500 calories alone. You're going to have to eat and eat and eat until you actually feel full.

> Do you see how easy it is to add 500 calories without even noticing it? It doesn't fill you up at all, so you wouldn't even be able to perceive it!

You know this to be true, don't you? Because those times you've decided to just have a little ice cream or cheese because it's "not that much" or "no big deal," you probably didn't stop there. It's not your fault, my friend. It's just that it takes such a large volume of calories in order to feel full on that kind of food. So it's not that you're ever choosing 500 calories of ice cream over 500 calories of salad. You're probably choosing 2000 calories of [fill in the blank] over 500 calories and a nice happy belly full of salad.

See how easy it is to get into trouble that way? And I'm not even talking about overall health concerns yet. That's a whole other level on top of this. At this moment, I'm strictly referring to weight loss as it's so powerfully connected to calorie density.

And then there's oil. Are you ready for this one? Take a big breath. Now let it out. It's going to be okay, just stay with me.

500 calories of oil is a mere drop in the bucket! Do you

see how easy it is to add 500 calories without even noticing it? It doesn't fill you up at all, so you wouldn't even be able to perceive it! You just drizzle on the calories without any additional satiation whatsoever. Eek!

Once you understand how calorie density works and what it feels like in your body, you can understand why the choices you've made in the past have created a history of being overweight. Remember that processed foods like bread and pasta fall very close to cheese in the calorie density chart. This means that if you're eating the diet that is common for most developed countries, you're eating a lot of animal products and processed foods, including bread and pasta and oil, and you're spending most of your time looking like the stomachs on the left - always scrounging around for more.

If you've been eating "normally" so far, as in eating the way most of us were raised, you've been filling your stomach at each meal with mostly meat, dairy, oil, and some veggies. This will have you taking in around 900-1,200 calories *per meal*. If you do that three times a day with snacks in between you will have been consuming so many calories that the only logical outcome is weight gain.

If you're anything like me, wanting to lose weight in the past, you've started doing things like restricting your portions, eliminating snacks, pushing yourself away from the table, drinking more water at meals, or any number of other tricks to try to *feel full on less food*.

The problem is, your stomach is designed to feel full. There is a whole cascade of chemical signals that control the hunger drive, turning it on and off. This is a fool-proof system designed hundreds of thousands of years ago in order to ensure the survival of the species. It's not to be taken lightly! One of those signals keeps driving you to eat until the stomach reaches a certain level of distension, or stretching out. When you're continually trying to override this switch, you're going to experience discomfort which some people call cravings. You're going to feel driven to eat, practically beyond your control.

You may be able to grit this out for a while, but eventually, your brain and body will win out, and you'll return to eating enough volume so that you feel full, regardless of the consequences. You'll convince yourself that it's crazy to starve (and it is) and so you'll just eat what you want. This is one of the reasons why people end up in yo-yo dieting cycles. You're constantly working against a very primal hunger mechanism that wants you to feel full, and it will eventually win!

The only types of food that fill your stomach with a reasonable or recommended amount of calories are vegetables, fruit, whole grains, and legumes. When you simply shift the kinds of foods you're eating toward the stomachs on the far right, you're going to be eating fewer calories and still feeling full. How amazing is that?

This is why your food choices matter when it comes to weight loss.

Any time I talk about calories, I just know someone out there is thinking, *"How about I just eat the cheese and the oil and work out more??"*

Yes, of course it matters how many calories you're burning, but do you know any exercise on the planet that can burn off an extra 1,500 to 2,000 calories?

You see, the average American consumes 3,600 calories per day, which is a significant excess for most women who could be doing very well eating 1,500 to 2,000 calories per day. Keeping up this trend will lead to steady weight gain month after month and year after year. You'd have to be doing some insane training in order to burn that many additional calories.

So what's more powerful: focusing on the fuel or the exercise?

Let's take two drastic examples of a gentle exercise versus a strenuous exercise.

EXERCISE	CALORIE BURN
Strolling at a slow pace for 10 minutes	75 calories
Stair climbing for 10 minutes	120 calories
Run up the stairs for 10 minutes	175 to 200 calories
*note: calorie burn varies per person and is related to your current weight.	

So from the easiest 10-minute exercise to the most strenuous 10-minute exercise, the calorie burn is just over double. Yet the calorie difference in a full stomach from the lowest calorie food to the highest calorie food is a 40 fold difference!

Let's translate that into numbers that you may be able to relate to better.

Let's just evaluate the decision to use a salad dressing

with oil vs a flavored balsamic vinegar with no oil. The veggies have filled you up, and the oil adds no extra bulk or satiety, so it doesn't fill you up any extra, but it does add an extra 500 calories.

So… in order to "burn off" the extra calories, you'd either have to stroll for 3 ½ hours or RUN up the stairs at a sustained pace for 30 minutes. That's just the choice between salad dressing or balsamic vinegar at a single meal. We didn't even get into throwing nuts and seeds on top, or heaven forbid, cheese!

And before you even start asking about the oils marketed as healthy… Hear this: when it comes to fat, oil is oil is oil. It all has 4,000 calories per pound. It's all 100% fat. There's just no escaping this fact. And just for extra ammunition, there's nothing about oil that's a "whole" food. It's strictly the fat component of a plant, isolated out and bottled up.

If you've got any concerns about excess weight, excess body fat, pre-diabetes, diabetes, high cholesterol, high blood pressure, erectile dysfunction, dementia, or stroke, then you'll want to stay away from oil.

I promised I wouldn't tell you what to do, right? You're a grown-up and you get to make your own choices. So when you ask me, *"Christin, but is it ok to have a little oil on my veggies? That's how I'm used to cooking them."*

I'll ask you, *"How long can you run up stairs without stopping?"*

Or, *"How quickly do you want to fit back into your pants?"*

Me, personally? I'd much rather just eat my food without oil, enjoy the heck out of it, put on my favorite jeans, and then go run up and down the stairs, or hike up a mountain, or chase my daughter on the playground just for fun!!

> Start filling up your plate with foods that are lower in calorie density. Do it for 30 days and see if what I'm saying is true for you

At the very least, just give it a try. Start filling up your plate with foods that are lower in calorie density. Do it for 30 days and see if what I'm saying is true for you. I've created my own tool to help you remember exactly what to eat.

Despite the fact that I've thrown around a lot of numbers and a lot of talk about calories, it was simply to give you a quantitative way to understand these principles at work. After today I hope we never talk about calories again! You don't need to remember any of the numbers. You'll understand why in the next chapter.

Fill Her Up, High Octane Please!

CLIENT SPOTLIGHT
MEET RISË (RHYMES WITH LISA)

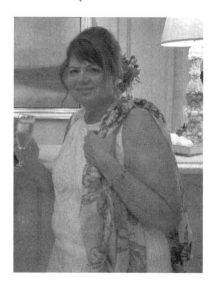
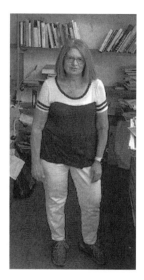
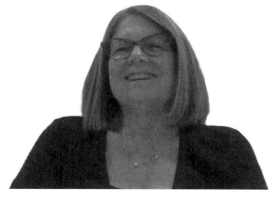

I've had a binge-eating disorder for as long as I can remember. I've tried every different diet I could get my hands on. You name it, I've tried it. I can tell you from experience the good news and the bad news: they all work until they don't.

I had even been WFPB (whole food plant-based) before joining The Forever Diet, but this was a lot more information for me and a whole lot more support. Not sure whether it would be any different from my past attempts, I followed the program religiously. I had NO idea how different the outcome would be, and I don't mean just in my waistline. I can't even tell you how different I am now, how much better I feel!

Before this program, I was totally frustrated with my mood, my frame of mind, and my anxiety. I didn't even realize it, but I think I was just grumpy all the time. All of it improved dramatically! I've been at it for almost a year now and everything keeps improving.

I have a lot on my plate. I'm a full-time caregiver to my elderly father. My husband had open-heart surgery right in the midst of COVID, and then our senior dog died. I don't know what would've happened if I didn't have this support. All I can say is that the old me would have been mopey and depressed and miserable.

But not the new me! Even with all of that on my plate, my food is fine! My binge eating is under control for the first time ever. I've lost so much weight even with everything that has been going on, it's really a miracle.

I still get into late-night snacking every once in a while, but it's not nearly as bad as it used to be, and I'm free of the guilt and torment I used to have. This has been the greatest gift - losing the guilt and shame I used to put myself through. When you have someone like Christin who's really there for you, and checks in with you to see how you're doing, it's a total gamechanger!

No matter what happened the day before, I get up in the morning and I'm right back on track.

> *I had no idea how much my food was affecting my mood. I had been so focused on weight loss that I completely overlooked the other effects of my food choices. Once I started following The Forever Diet methods, everything changed. I felt better quickly, and then the weight fell off shortly after. I'm so thankful that I set aside past experiences and approached this with an open mind! I hope you can too. I'm rooting for you!*
>
> ~RISË

READY, SET, ACTION! NOW IT'S YOUR TURN FOR RESULTS!

What was your biggest takeaway when it comes to calorie density? What is it that you wish to remember the next time you're faced with a temptation, or you're deciding what to put on your plate? Record it here:

_____

_____

_____

If you've been relying on exercise to "burn off" extra calories, or to punish yourself for overeating, or in order to justify eating something decadent, how do you see that differently now? Write it in your own words to anchor it in.

_____

_____

If you've learned about calorie density before but have had trouble implementing it consistently, how can you up your game a bit?

_____

_____

Bonus points for sharing your takeaways in the Facebook group!

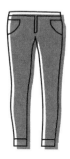

CHAPTER 5:

Green Means GO!

*If you quit now, you'll end up right where you first began.
And when you first began,
you were desperate to be where you are now.
Don't quit! Keep going!*

~ ANONYMOUS

I promised you good news, and here it is. The good news is you are not about to be spending the remainder of your days living off of cardboard and carrots and iceberg lettuce. YAY!

I know that can feel like the default sometimes when you're new to this and it feels like *everything* is off-limits. To make it super easy for you, I developed a tool to explain what to eat in order to really cut down on your confusion and streamline your decision-making. Following this system will absolutely help you slim down almost regardless of the portions of food you eat.

If you find yourself constantly wandering to the kitchen out of stress or boredom, THIS is the system that will save you. It's a way to look at calorie density in terms of 3 categories, green light, yellow light, and red light. Understanding calorie density by the number is useful, but you don't have to memorize any numbers in order to succeed. If you can refer to this chart, you'll have everything you need to know! It applies calorie density to the real world.

First and foremost, green means GO!

These are foods you can eat as much as you want, anytime you want, with very few exceptions! You want to be eating these foods: leafy greens, vegetables, starches, legumes, whole grains, and fruit to the point where you are satiated and full at the end of your meal, but not uncomfortably stuffed. It may take some time to tune into and to trust your hunger signals again, so grant yourself some grace as you make this transition.

Green Means GO!

Green Light
CHEAT SHEET

GREEN LIGHT FOODS
No Limits! The More the Merrier

All leafy greens: Spinach, bok choy, kale, collards, romaine. cabbage, etc

All vegetables: Bell peppers, red beets, tomatoes, carrots, broccoli, cauliflower, celery, zucchini eggplant, onions, mushrooms, etc

Starches: Potatoes, sweet potatoes, squashes, plantains etc

Legumes: Lentils (all colors), chickpeas, black beans, pinto beans, kidney beans, mung beans

Whole Grains: Brown rice, quinoa, oats, millet, amaranth, etc

Fruit: Apples, oranges, plantains, strawberries, raspberries, kiwi, blueberries, grapes, blackberries, melon, cherries, bananas, and more

Preparations: Raw, steamed, boiled, roasted, or air-fried are all perfectly fine!

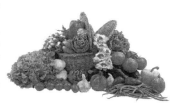

YELLOW LIGHT FOODS
Proceed with Caution. These foods are all calorically dense.

Nuts and Nut Butters

Coconut

Seeds (includes seed bread & crackers)

Avocado

Dried Fruit

Tofu, Tempeh

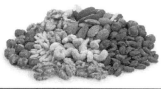

RED LIGHT FOODS:
These Foods Do Not Serve You! Stay Away!

All animal products: If it walks, flies, swims, or has a mother, let it be. That is, meat, fish, birds, eggs, or dairy.

All oils: coconut, olive, canola, vegetable, flax seed, grape seed, etc. This includes anything deep fried, cooked in oil, or with oil listed in the ingredients.

All highly processed foods: sugar, flour, alcohol, or products made with them.

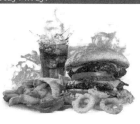

Figure 3: Green Light Cheat Sheet

This is not a complete list of every single fruit, vegetable, and starch available to you, but it does give you a great list to start with. You'll have an opportunity at the end of the chapter to brainstorm some more of your favorites that may not be shown here.

LEAFY GREENS

In the Green section of the chart, you will find that we start with the king of nutrition, the leafy greens! I can't emphasize enough how important it is to have leafy greens in your diet daily, and preferably multiple times a day. Many of my clients have experienced a huge leap in their success when they began increasing their intake of greens, and many now eat a sweet cinnamon-sprinkled version of greens and beans for breakfast! It sounds strange, I know, but so does resigning to be heavy, unhealthy, and unhappy when there's a perfectly wonderful alternative!

VEGETABLES

I'm sure you already know that it's great to eat your vegetables, and I won't argue. But be warned, you can't live on veggies alone!

I know many people who have tried to do this. Rather than following a system like this one, they were trying to apply old dieting principles of portion control and caloric restriction to a whole food plant-based diet, and it simply doesn't work well. That's one of the perks of this system. You don't have to practice restriction and portion control!

I have a friend who tried desperately to lose weight by going vegan. She was eating carrot sticks and celery sticks, some hummus, and a lot of Diet Coke mixed in with some soy caramel lattes. That was pretty much it. She didn't take the time to create a balanced diet, and it backfired.

Yes, she did lose weight for a while. But she wasn't getting nearly enough nutrients from her very limited food and was constantly hungry from not eating enough volume. She was irritable from always being hungry, and she was puzzled by how I could eat such a "limited" diet. I was bouncing off the walls with energy, and she was only remaining upright because of the caffeine and sugar.

In addition to the caffeine and sugar problem, she was experiencing such a difficult time because she had one toe in this diet and nine toes in dieting the old fashioned way - portion control. The latter relies on a tremendous amount of willpower and is not destined to last. So after she tried for a while, she gave up on going vegan and went back to her old habits. In record time, she regained all of the weight she had lost and written off veganism as a failure.

You cannot live on veggies alone, so please don't try this in an attempt to speed up your weight loss. It is not sustainable and is likely to land you right back where you started! You'll be severely under-eating calories and you won't have the satiating starches to fill the rest of your nutrient needs and to keep you going.

STARCHES

So here's the chance you've been waiting for: Carb loading. I joke about being a carb-aholic, and I suppose it's not unfounded, but it's worth noting that there are many different kinds of carbohydrates. As the Green Light Cheat Sheet lays out, this is your opportunity to go ahead and fill up on the starches like potatoes, sweet potatoes, and squashes.

> As the Green Light Cheat Sheet lays out, this is your opportunity to go ahead and fill up on the starches like potatoes, sweet potatoes, and squashes

But don't stop there! Also pile up the legumes like black beans, chickpeas, kidney beans, and lentils. Beans are your new best friends as they're a wonderful little package containing protein, carbohydrates, and even a little fat, in just the right proportion. Enjoy whole grains like brown rice, quinoa, oat groats, steel-cut oats, millet, amaranth, etc, and all sorts of fruit! Choose from strawberries, raspberries, kiwis, blueberries, plantains, blackberries, melon, cherries, and bananas, just to name a few.

By now, you may be wondering, "*Hey Christin, how do I*

prepare or eat these things?"

Well, you can eat them raw, steamed, boiled, canned, roasted, or air fried. All of those are perfectly fine. The only thing to stay away from is any preparation that requires oil.

If you need help cooking without oil, I can help you with that. All you need to do is have a little liquid and a little patience with learning something new. Keep water or broth handy by the stove, and add a little at a time as things start to stick to the pan. Keep the heat to medium or medium- high, and you'll have an easier time producing tasty meals without burning or having a sticky mess.

So those are your Green Light foods - leafy greens, veggies, legumes, grains, and fruit. Green means go, got it?

The Yellow Light category is one that gets the most people into trouble so this is the one I want to make sure you understand. This is where we put those foods that are natural, as in unprocessed, but they are richer and higher in calories than anything you'll find in the Green Light area. *Some people* can eat them without any problems whatsoever while *most people* cannot eat them in unlimited quantities and still lose weight. If you're overweight, there's a good chance you're in the category of *most people* and would benefit from limiting or avoiding these foods, at least for the first month or two. These things aren't off-limits forever, but until you can bring your weight and your lab work to where you want it, and you've maintained it for some time, it's a good idea to shy away from this category or start to wean yourself away from it.

It's worth noting that this category is great for children

or the elderly or for endurance athletes who need to gain or maintain weight (assuming they don't already have heart disease or diabetes). These are perfectly healthy foods that offer many benefits. It's just that their consumption needs to be moderated for most of us, and they can lead down a rocky road.

Included are things like nuts and nut butters, coconut, seeds, avocado, dried fruit, tofu, and tempeh, and instant oats.

As an added bonus, many people experience great freedom from food cravings when they avoid the Yellow Light category for a while. If it's too much for you to even attempt right now, don't sweat it! We'll talk more about that in the next chapter.

Every individual is different, and this is where we usually see a lot of differences. These foods may be fine for those people who don't have any trouble moderating or limiting quantities. Take my husband for example, who can eat 1 Brazil nut every 3 days. Or he could open a jar of almond butter, eat one teaspoon, and put the rest back for months. I have no idea how he does that! For me, I might intend to eat one ounce of fresh, unsalted raw nuts a day, but by the fifth day, I'd be stopping at the gas station to grab a big bag of salty, oil-roasted nuts convincing myself I really need them for the healthy fats…

Simply take the yellow for what it is - a sign of caution - and do with it what you will. I've seen way too many people fail and not reach their goals simply because they couldn't moderate the Yellow Light foods. So if you have a hunch that's you, it probably is. Try laying off it for a while and see what happens. It's just a temporary experiment.

Now, for the Red Light area, I'm going to make this super easy for you. Just picture the red light district in Amsterdam, and that'll help you remember you'll find some scary things here that do not serve you! Stay away from them! Run away, don't even look back over your shoulder!

It's time to address the elephant in the room. The Red Light area is where the animal products fit in. If it walks, flies, swims, or has a mother, it does *not* belong on your plate. So that includes all meat, fish, birds, eggs, and dairy.

If you're eating meat, fish, and dairy now, please don't freak out. I know that this will be a big change for you. But let me ask, "*Are you looking for big results or teeny-tiny results?*"

I don't subscribe to the "no pain, no gain" approach to life. But I do know that if you keep doing what you've always done, you'll keep getting what you've always had. My aim here is to make the *results* way more enticing than the changes.

Let me share with you exactly what happened when I started eating this way.

If you recall, my doctor had given me 6 months to correct my high blood pressure with lifestyle changes. Or else. He told me I'd have to start taking medication if I didn't turn things around in that time. "Some people just have bad genes," he reassured me, as I was walking out of the office.

After 4 weeks of eating a whole food plant-based diet just as I've described to you so far, my headaches disappeared. I was having headaches 3-4 days a week. I didn't even realize how normal they were for me until they were gone!

I started to feel better. I had more energy. I used to collapse on the couch after work and my husband would have to poke and prod me to get me up to go to bed, but I quit falling asleep during the day completely. I used to have a habit of falling asleep in the car as soon as we went anywhere and I didn't have to drive. That stopped immediately.

My seasonal allergies virtually disappeared for the first time in my life. I was never expecting that, but it was my experience and I've since learned of so many people who have similar results.

> I knew beyond the shadow of a doubt that I had the power to outrun my family's terrible health history

Honestly, I didn't even know how crappy I was feeling until I started feeling better. I knew something good was going on, and I couldn't wait any longer to check my progress. I got my lab work done and went back to the doc in 1 month instead of 6. I was beaming with pride when he took my blood pressure this time. It had dropped from 140/90 to 120/72.

BOOM!

My cholesterol and other markers all slid right down into the normal zone. My pants were looser too, and for the first time in my life, I knew beyond the shadow of a

Green Means GO!

doubt that I had the power to outrun my family's terrible health history. And I was doing it without a lick of exercise.

I had done it by adjusting what was on my plate. I chose normal, tasty, clean food from the Green Light area, and it wasn't even that hard, especially once I got through the first few weeks of transition. Food really is medicine and I was taking on a double dose!

Wanna hear something crazy though? My doctor looked over my results with only mild enthusiasm. He wasn't nearly as impressed as he should have been. And eventually said, *"Some people just have good genes. Guess you're one of them!"*

Wait. What?!

Did he just say that? I thought he said I had bad genes. Did they change in the last month?

That statement changed my life forever. It became crystal clear right then and there: I am the only one looking out for me, and it's my responsibility (and privilege) to do what's best for my body! So I set out to do exactly that.

> I am the only one looking out for me, and it's my responsibility (and privilege) to do what's best for my body!

During that first 30 day experiment, everything changed for me. It did feel a little challenging at the time, but it was completely doable. I was just eating real food, after all! There wasn't anything crazy about it. It was just different than what I was used to.

For the first week or so I dropped all of the animal products. Once I had learned about oils and their fat content, and their role in heart disease and diabetes, it was easy to cut them out, too.

You'll see in the Red Light area that it's best to steer clear of highly processed food like sugar, flour, and alcohol, and products made from them. Their calorie density is far too high for comfort, and they don't serve your body well in any way.

I'll be explaining more about how to put together meals that make sense, but for now, stock up on some groceries to have Green Light food on hand in your kitchen. That's a really great start!

Green Means GO!

CLIENT SPOTLIGHT
MEET TAMMIEBETH

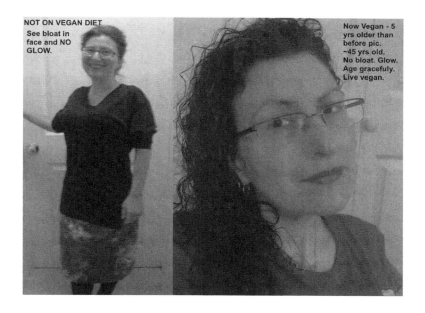

My friends would probably say that I've had a healthy diet and lifestyle for quite some time now. In fact, I cut out meat and dairy back in 1989 when I fell in love with the concept of a vegetarian diet during my Nutrition class at University. However, it took me some time to learn to eat a healthy unprocessed diet. When I learned about the health and power available to us in fruits and veggies, boy did I go unprocessed - in fact, I went raw/vegan for a year or two around 2000.

I was following people like David Wolfe, Erik Markus, and John Robbins long before *Forks Over Knives* came on the scene. Cooking and eating healthy has always been a big part of my life and I actually published several cookbooks covering everything from introducing your children to raw foods to cooking vegan when your family is not, without spending all day in the kitchen making multiple meals. I just loved sharing my passion for health with others! This led to over a decade helping others as a health coach.

Over the years I got off track a few times with either processed or non-Vegan foods and had to self-correct. Contradicting studies would make me doubt my own knowledge and experience. After a one year deviation away from a Plant-Based Diet, I earned a certification from E-Cornell in Plant-Based Nutrition so I would never be shaken by a bad study or marketing again!

Fast forward several years, I saw Christin's program. I'm always looking to learn and grow, and so even though I already had a wealth of knowledge, I wanted to hear what she had to say. I wouldn't have even thought it was possible for it to CHANGE MY LIFE SO MUCH, but it did!!

I thought I knew how to be my best, and make the best choices for myself, but when I heard it explained in The Forever Diet programs, something totally clicked that I had never even realized was missing up until that point!

All of a sudden my 'why' became crystal clear. I identified small things that I was doing (or not doing) that were keeping me from being my best self.

When I started the challenge, I felt like my diet was already clean and I also had plant-based education, decades of experience and followed the brightest minds in the movement, but I still had massive breakthroughs! I streamlined my time in the kitchen and my food, I made mental shifts that increased my joy each day, and I learned how to make my home like a spa and truly enjoy it. I also learned more about the biology behind *why* this works. Christin does an amazing job of taking information from many places and condensing it down to bite sized pieces full of useful take-always.

I have completely changed my daily routines so that I'm spending less time in the kitchen than ever before. I've integrated the Forever Diet recipes and principles into my life. It now makes up pretty much ALL of what I eat and how I approach life! Bonus: during this time I went through menopause with nary a symptom! I feel amazing and as far as food, I have all the flavors and textures I need… so why would I change?

The people in the group are fantastic. I totally found my tribe. Now you can find me active in the group sharing recipes and experiences. Every day I get excited watching new people come into the program because I know what lies in store for them and I know the potential that they have with such rich tools and support at their fingertips. I wish every single person I know would consider joining this program! Our society would be transformed to be healthier and happier, and so would our planet.

> *It's not always easy to make changes, but it's always worth it! Don't let any more time pass you by. You deserve to feel better immediately! Take the time to figure out where would be the best place to start, and just start!*
>
> ~TAMMIEBETH

READY, SET, ACTION

Okay, it's time to get to work!

- [ ] Hop over to the resource page at www.theforeverdiet.org/book-bonuses and grab your printable copy of the Green Light Cheat Sheet. Review it and hang it up in your kitchen for easy reference.

- [ ] Identify 3-6 foods in the Red Light area that might be the most problematic for you. This is not to scold you but rather to help you shine the light on where you could make the biggest impact with the least amount of change.

Write them here and make a commitment to eliminate them. You pick the foods. You pick your time frame. The only directive is to decide.

_____

_____

_____

_____

_____

_____

I'll eliminate these foods for the next 30 days starting on:

_____

☐ Identify 6-8 foods in the Green Light area that you'd like to eat more often. Choose foods you already like and are familiar with. If you don't have enough of those, simply brainstorm new foods you're willing to try!

_____
_____
_____
_____
_____
_____

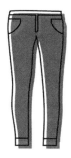

CHAPTER 6

Kicking Cravings to the Curb

We are all a little broken. That's how the light gets in.
~ERNEST HEMINGWAY

How many times have you committed to a diet or a lifestyle change, setting out with so much motivation and determination, only to wind up right back where you started? Sometimes the gusto lasts for weeks, sometimes it's a matter of days, and sometimes it's only a few hours before we're right back to old habits. It can be exhausting and downright depressing to give in to cravings when we "know better" and truly want to make better decisions. We often beat ourselves up for being "weak" and chalk up the attempt to one more failure. If this scenario is all too familiar, then please take comfort in knowing that you're not alone and also that the solution is about to appear.

As humans, we are very susceptible to cravings, and they're constantly pulling us off course. You might do great for a while, but when faced with the temptations at a restaurant, or a friend's house, or a wedding, you find yourself dabbling with a few bites here and there. Next thing you know, several days have gone by, weeks start to pass, and what began as "just this once" turns into a full-blown all-you-can-eat buffet, and you're right back to old habits.

Once you understand what's really going on, you'll be able to master yourself and overcome cravings once and for all.

It all boils down to survival, evolution, and calorie density. Let me explain.

Our ancestors were born into an era of food scarcity and an environment that lacked accessible and reliable sources of energy. The greatest threat to their survival was starvation. Let me say that again - the folks who came before you had one major threat to their survival and it was not heart disease, diabetes, nor cancer. It was starvation. Lack of sufficient calories. Not enough to eat. In a nutshell: their problems were way different than modern-day problems. And yet we're still trying to solve these problems with the same brains they had.

So in the times of dire food scarcity, the ones who survived long enough to reproduce were the ones who were better at finding food. They developed a keen memory for the location of food sources which helped them to stay well fed. Have you ever realized what a keen memory you have for food sources? Even when you try to hide something from yourself, you can never actually forget it's there, right? What about your favorite restaurants? Couldn't you practically drive there in your sleep? Is it easy to picture your favorite meals? To recall the smell of your mom's best casserole or gran's favorite cookies? These memories are so easy to recall, and it's because our ancestors relied upon this skill for survival. It was such a crucial adaptation for survival, it became powerfully engrained in generations to follow.

Find food. Remember where it is. Come back for more.

But it wasn't just a matter of finding any food. It had to be the best food. You see, in order to get the best *fuel* to sustain their physical activity, they sought the most calories for the least amount of effort. They had to choose the biggest bang for their buck because surely it wouldn't make sense to walk for 5 miles to munch on leaves, fruit, and bark. That would mean expending 500 calories only to consume 200 calories. That's not advanced nutrition science, that's simple math, and getting it right led them to the survival solution.

Back in their day, berries, fruits, and roots (aka potatoes) were really good finds! Leafy greens, grasses, and other low-calorie foods were edible but didn't provide nearly as much energy. In order to ensure survival, the human brain was guided by a feedback mechanism that would predictably motivate the human to choose one food over another. This trick was critical in allowing humans to live long enough to procreate and further the species.

In short, they were operating on the principles of calorie density, looking for the most calorically dense food, with the least amount of effort. But how could our ancestors tell the difference in calorie density without any modern scales or fancy measurement devices or my handy dandy chart?

When they ate something high in calorie density, their brain released dopamine, a neurotransmitter known as the "feel-good hormone." The greater the calorie density of a particular food, the greater the amount of dopamine released.

Dopamine makes you feel good! More dopamine makes you feel *fantastic*!

Just like the pleasure-seeking humans we are today, our early ancestors were guided by this mechanism. It led them to repeatedly seek and find the most calorie-rich food because that's what had the greatest potential to sustain life. As a result, they were predictably drawn to eat fruit, nuts, seeds, and veggies. They ate some meat because it was by far the most calorie-dense food in the environment. It certainly wasn't obtained easily though. It took massive effort to secure those calories, so out of necessity, they only ate it sparingly.

Human brains became incredibly proficient at running the cost-benefit analysis of various food sources. It was a matter of life and death and it became an equation any of them could run in a fraction of a second, subconsciously.

So this is a good thing, right? Our brains learned how to find *healthy* food to keep us alive. Our ancestors survived long enough to give us life, so something was going right. That should serve us well, but there's one major problem. Our brains did not evolve to find healthy food. Our brains evolved to find the *richest* food in any environment. In an environment where the richest foods are nuts, seeds, and berries, the organism is likely to thrive using this mechanism.

However, in a modern environment where the richest food includes deep-fried candy bars, donuts, and double bacon cheeseburgers, the organism is in BIG trouble. We're practically doomed for failure. If you look around at your fellow modern humans, you know this to be true.

So what happens today when you follow your biological instinct and reach for the richest food in your environment? You get a huge hit of dopamine, and it feels good! No wonder you keep reaching for it. Everything in your biology is telling you to go grab it and shove it in your mouth quickly before someone else does. Do you think you can just ignore that? Think again. The dopamine cascade affects the same pleasure center of the brain as sex and even cocaine and other narcotics. When you have a little, it only makes you want more. Uh oh.

This is why it's virtually impossible to ignore the call of the Oreo! Or bread or candy, or chips and french fries. Even though the availability of highly processed food is relatively recent, our ancient brains remember well where to find the richest food, and it keeps calling us back over and over again.

> The dopamine cascade affects the same pleasure center of the brain as sex and even cocaine and other narcotics. When you have a little, it only makes you want more.

If you think about the foods that most often throw you off track, I would venture to guess that they're particularly high in sugar, fat, and salt. These (particularly oils and refined sugars) are some of the most processed and therefore most calorically dense food-like substances we have available. They're also staples in the Standard American Diet which has spread just as destructively as wildfire. The ongoing consumption of processed foods is one of the main reasons so many people are struggling to lose weight.

When you consume them, it begins the dopamine cascade and you're reinforced for this behavior which will only perpetuate it. Give in to one small craving and you'll just keep wanting more. Deny yourself the food you're craving and the pull may become even more intense before it begins to fade.

What happens when you commit (again) to reach for healthier food, which is much lower in calorie density?

You've read the books, you understand the science, and you know it's what your body really needs. You start eating salads, vegetables, and potatoes, healthy whole natural food that your body was intended to use as fuel. You're filling up on greens and other things that are high in nutrients while low in caloric density. Does it *feel* good?

NOPE! Not at first.

You get a very low hit of dopamine and you get the chemical signal that it wasn't the best decision. Your brain pulls a temper tantrum trying to get its way, and you experience cravings. The only logical step is to wander to the kitchen where you have snacks in the pantry, novelties in the freezer, and restaurant leftovers in the fridge. They're full of sugar, oil, and salt, and other red light ingredients. You are automatically drawn to them. Should you decide to indulge and eat some of those "treats", you get that big hit of dopamine, and it will feel good. So you will keep eating it. And then you'll feel full and then overfull and then *wham*!

Guilt sets in.

You feel bloated and uncomfortable and then you feel guilty because once again you have fallen prey to cravings. You feel weak. You feel annoyed with yourself, disappointed with yourself, and then what always happens?

If you're like most of us, you say *the hell with it*! You throw up your hands and decide to start again on Monday. You've already screwed up. You might as well get rid of all the junk in the house, so you eat it all as quickly as possible!

Am I right?

What I hope you're starting to hear is it's not your fault that you've struggled with this. Our food supply is artificially high in fat and sugar and salt and it has hijacked your brain to the point where it's virtually impossible to override the drive to eat rich, calorie-dense foods.

So, that begs the question....

How do you lose weight in a modern environment?

There are two choices.

One option is that you attempt to eat "everything in moderation," and use portion control so you don't eat too much of the "bad stuff." Remember the discussion about the stomachs being only partially full of meat, cheese, oil, and processed foods? The fatal flaw in that plan is that your stomach wants to feel full. Whatever you choose to eat, you will likely receive the signals to keep eating until your stomach is physically full and partially distended. Because the hunger drive is controlled by a complex cascade of signaling hormones, eating to a point where you're less than full requires a massive, superhuman amount of willpower.

Think about it - how long would humans have lasted if we had no idea when to eat and when to stop? This is a primal instinct and it won't be overridden without a fight. Nor should it! If you're really determined, you may be able to gut it out for a while, but it won't last. We know this to be true because the entire dieting industry is built upon this fact. You can try to restrict portions for a while, and even though you may get short-term results with this method, you won't be able to keep it up forever. Eventually, something will cross your path to throw you off course and you'll be back to where you started.

The other option is changing the *type of food* you put in your body. Avoid the calorically dense foods and focus on filling up with foods that are high in nutrients instead. The more consistently you do that, the more quickly you'll be recreating the diet that is natural for humans. Even though your initial cravings may show up something fierce, this will only last a very short while. You'll navigate the detox and you'll be all the better for it! You'll be experiencing a host of health benefits, you'll lose excess fat, you'll have more energy, and you'll start feeling younger every day! The most wonderful benefit is that within a matter of days (or sometimes weeks), your cravings will dissipate.

Now, often people ask me, "*What about natural sugar? Zero-calorie sweeteners? Which kind of sugar is best?*" Here's an important thing to understand about sugar. Processed sugar includes everything from high fructose corn syrup to cane sugar to maple syrup, honey, agave, Stevia, and yes even the next artificial/natural sweetener that gets released on the market. And the one after that!

When it comes to cravings, and when it comes to brain chemistry, sugar is sugar. When you have a little, your brain calls for more and it won't let up until it gets it. And even then, it wants more after that. The only way around that is to consume sugar as it is found in whole foods - fresh or frozen fruit. That's the only place you'll find it packaged with the fiber that makes it safe to consume.

Ready to kick the cravings monster to the curb for good? Eat real food: vegetables, fruits, starches, whole grains, legumes, and eventually some nuts and seeds. It is as simple as that. If you want to find Easy Street and succeed with a healthy lifestyle, the very quickest way to get there is to shift from eating a lot of processed foods to a lot of whole foods. In following the principles of calorie density and eating food in the Green Light and Yellow Light areas, you'll be well on your way to solving this mystery while working with your natural brain chemistry and not against it.

When you are ready to make changes to the type of food you put in your body, there are two ways to do it.
- All at once
- Gradually

If you're an all-or-nothing person, then you'll do better ripping the band-aid off and going all-in. Go ahead and clean out your pantry to whatever degree you can. Remove the junk foods from your house or at least separate them for your normal food supply. Begin to eat all of your foods from the Green Light Area, and stick with that for 14-30 days before introducing Yellow Light foods.

You will likely have a few uncomfortable days in the beginning, but you'll get through the physical detox quite quickly, and then you'll be well on your way to calmer waters. You will elicit that calm brain quickly and you start to reset your palate as well. These two factors will help you crush your cravings rapidly.

If you're a dip-your-toe-in-the-water type of person, then you'll do best taking the changes gradually. Using the Green-Light Cheat Sheet, and the Calorie Density Chart, see where you can add in more of the healthier options. Maybe you start with a Green Light breakfast, and then you eat the regular lunches and dinners you're used to. Or maybe you start adding in a small serving of vegetables before each meal. Or perhaps you switch to a giant salad as the main meal one a day. Do this for a week, and then the next week you can bite off a new change.

Taking the process slowly may make the cravings persist a bit longer because you'll be continually rewarded with a dopamine hit every time you eat something rich. However, there are many people for whom this is the right way to go. If you tend to be so perfectionist in your approach, then perhaps this is an exercise for you to take it slowly and see how you do.

Only you know yourself, and you may eventually try both methods. There's no wrong way to take action except to take no action.

As for the remainder of your education, we're not done yet! Give yourself about a week to soak in each of the remaining chapters. You'll be highly successful as long as you continue the education and stay tuned in for support. We've talked a lot about food so far so that you can understand the mechanics of what's at play, and the next chapter will really bring home some of the issues that a lot of people get tripped up on. After that, we're going to go deep into some factors way beyond the food, and once you have those skills under your belt, look out! Success is all but inevitable.

Be sure to join my private Facebook group in order to

ask your questions and get support from other people sharing experiences and overcoming similar struggles.

It doesn't matter whether you want to go all-in or just dip your toe in the water. You can make changes quickly or you can make them slowly. Just be sure to keep at it consistently and take advantage of the education and support you have available to help you stick to it.

Regardless of how you implement, keep moving slow and steady with the education piece. This is a practice and an art. It's not a flip-the-switch-once-you-read-the-magic-book type of program! You've got to actually DO the work too. What we're about to embark upon - ripping free from the grip of constant cravings - can be a difficult thing to do. It can also be the most freeing thing you've ever done. It's worth it!

But just like an alcoholic trying to ditch the bottle, you don't want to go it alone. Find your tribe in the Facebook group, keep them close, and let's do this together!

You're probably wondering, "*How do you know what's actually a whole food anyway? The packaging and labeling can be so confusing.*" I'm so glad you asked! I'll cover that in the next chapter to squash the confusion.

Kicking Cravings to the Curb

CLIENT SPOTLIGHT
MEET LINDSEY

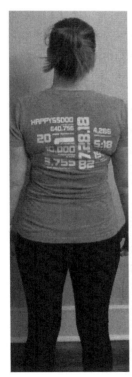
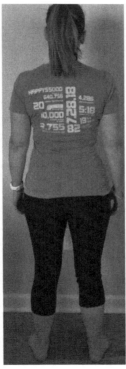
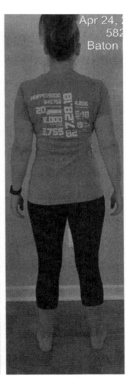

Having been an athlete all my life and understanding the ways to get in shape and healthy (or so I thought); I didn't think I had much to learn about nutrition. I wanted to get fit again after experiencing highs and lows of weight loss after having a child at 31. I didn't have much weight to lose, but I knew I could make huge improvements with the right program. I planned to start CrossFit. I started learning about the importance of food and focused on their strong push for eating a Paleo lifestyle as I continued with their workouts.

My reason for trying CrossFit started out as the vanity of getting back to a weight I was comfortable with and fitting in my clothes, but I also wanted to be healthier. After I didn't see enough results with intense CrossFit workouts and Paleo, I learned enough to know that I wanted to try going plant-based. My transition to plant-based eating was slow. I tried multiple times on my own for 2 years without meat or dairy. But it just wasn't working well for me. I don't give up easily, so I began signing up for every free plant-based guide I could find. I tried some recipes, but I just didn't have a clear plan to execute or time to learn all of the "new" ingredients and how to prep them without becoming stuck in the kitchen all day. And then finally...

I found Baby Got Back In Her Pants and I decided to try it.

I was initially skeptical because I had already learned so much, but it wasn't clicking. Through watching her videos and getting personal insights, I started to trust what she was saying and lean in for another shot! With all the knowledge I was gaining, Christin also had the motivation *and* the 'how to' I needed, and it was a game-changer! The new methods provided me with an understanding of exactly *how* to make the changes in my diet, and why. I successfully moved away from dairy and oil completely for the first time and I was *shocked* at what a difference it made! I lost 10 pounds just from removing oil. I couldn't even believe how easy it was once I knew what to replace it with and how to cook without it!

After the initial scale numbers stopped dropping, the changes in my body were still dramatically continuing. I kept getting leaner and more toned. I was seeing results in *weeks* that I hadn't seen in a year of CrossFit! I could be certain it was the food, as my workouts are not at all intense.

I don't know when it happened, but I moved on from caring about weight to my overall health. Now, I don't have to work out nearly as much to maintain the same fitness level and I recover much faster. I can feel the difference in my muscles and joints after dropping oil and sugar out of my diet. I jog a couple of miles a day and that's it. With the food I eat now, I can take off for a run after breakfast instead of feeling lazy and stuffed. I know it's hard to understand until you feel it for yourself, but I can now say for myself - I just feel better, stronger, and more clear than ever!

With each progress picture, I keep expecting my progress to stop, but the improvements keep on coming with minimal effort! I can see more definition in every photo, and it has been so rewarding to finally see everything come together! If I'd seen my own Before and After pictures somewhere else, I might doubt they're even real, but I can vouch for it! This really is me, and I'm grateful to be able to share!!

> *I tried to do this on my own for 2 years, and all of the resources I had found just left me confused and I never made any progress. After using Christin's methods, everything really clicked for me. I was so ready to go all-in, and I'm never looking back. I can't wait to hear if the same is true for you! There's only one way to find out!*
>
> ~LINDSEY

READY, SET, ACTION!

Ok, now it's your turn! There are a lot of different ways to succeed, and the first step is to decide which approach you're going to take. Are you ready to go all-in, or are you ready to dip your toe in the water? Be honest here. Which method is most likely to be successful for you?

- [ ] I'm all in!
- [ ] I'm dipping my toe in!
- [ ] Commit to 1 meal a day
  Which meal will it be? _____

OK good! Now that we've got that squared away, here's your assignment for this chapter. For those all-in folks, head to the resource page: www.theforeverdiet.org/book-bonuses and download the 3-Day Detox. The instructions should be self-explanatory, but feel free to ask any questions in the Facebook Group. We'll be happy to guide you!

For the dipping a toe folks, here's your project. Choose one meal a day that you can start making a Green Light meal. Breakfast is often the easiest place to start because we're typically at home, in the most control of the choices. But that's not the case for everyone. So choose what it is for you. Choose one meal a day to eat exclusively from the Green Light foods.

Do this for a whole week, and check in with us to share how it's going. After you're feeling pretty comfortable with this, try adding a second meal.

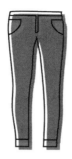

CHAPTER 7

If Only Pasta Grew on Trees

You don't have to cook fancy or complicated masterpieces - just good food from fresh ingredients.

~ JULIA CHILD

I'm going to hand you a framework to make food decisions going forward. If you have felt confused by all the "eat this, not that" talk you've seen in various places, or all of the claims on packaging about low fat this, and whole grain that, then this is for you. At the end of this chapter, you're going to understand exactly what I mean when I refer to a *whole food* vs processed food.

Eating a "plant-based" diet can have a few different interpretations, varying from eating mostly plants but some animals, to eating strictly vegan, with a lot of variations in between. On the other hand, though, eating a Whole Food Plant-Based diet has a very specific definition: which is: Eating a diet made up exclusively of whole plant foods such as vegetables, whole grains, legumes, and fruit.

It also implies avoiding all animal products. Last I checked, animals were not plants, so…. That's already included in the definition.

It also means avoiding processed foods because they are, by definition, not whole. Let's go ahead and dive into this part more. This is where most people get confused or thrown off track, and today is the day we can fix that.

There's at least some universal agreement that things like donuts, candy bars, and corn curls are processed. But what about things like whole grain crackers, whole grain bread, lentil pasta? It starts to get fuzzy, doesn't it? The growing list of "healthy" products (products being the key word) and their impressive labels is partially to blame for massive confusion.

So rather than discuss what's processed, let's ask a different question.

"*Is it a whole food?*"

Here's the secret, the surefire way to tell: Look at a food item and ask yourself, "*Does this still look like it did when it was growing?*"

Let's take these few examples: peppers, carrots, bananas.

Do they look like something you would see growing on a bush or in a tree? Of course! Dig in!

Okay, that was just a warm-up. How about these: lentils, brown rice, quinoa, chickpeas?

Yep! These are all whole foods, looking quite like they would right after being harvested! Sure, you'd want to cook them or sprout them before eating them, but they sure do look exactly like they did when they were harvested.

Here's where it gets tricky, and here's where my definition is going to make a massive difference in your pants size! How about these?

Whole grain bread, seed crackers, or pasta...

Do these items still look like they were just picked off a bush or a tree? No, not quite...

Have you ever actually seen a pasta tree?

Yes, they came from whole foods at one point, but they are no longer. The grains were harvested, processed into flour, and then made into different products. There's a whole spectrum of processing, but in every case, the original whole food has been modified in such a way that it no longer gets digested the same way the original whole food would be digested. That's what matters.

What happens in your body is different because of the processing. In almost all cases, the fiber has been stripped away. So what was once a perfectly healthy, whole, natural food, is no longer recognizable to your eyes, nor to your body.

Now, back to your waistline for a second. Remember that lesson on calorie density? It's about to all make even more sense now!

Let's take a specific example - corn kernels. Perfectly healthy food, right? But as it gets processed and made into different products, watch how the calorie density goes up with each level of processing.

½ cup of corn	60 calories
½ cup of corn flour	210 calories
1 cup of corn tortilla chips (15-20 chips)	300 calories
1 corn muffin	420 calories
½ cup of corn oil	1,000 calories

Remember, as the calorie density goes up, you're taking in more calories and you're feeling less full. Now that you understand calorie density and whole food vs processed foods, can you see why you may be struggling with weight loss?

If you had to create a formula for weight gain, this is what it would look like - eat as much processed food as possible. Eat as much as possible in the Red Light area, and make sure it's heavily processed. That's the only way you can consume the astronomical amount of calories that is making so many of us overweight, obese, and feeling miserable.

And what about fruit juice? It seems healthy enough. It is, after all, made only from fruit, right? Unfortunately, there's a problem that's really easy to overlook. So let's look at that for a second. If you ate an average-sized orange, you'd have about 1 cup of orange sections. That would give you about 60 calories, including 12 g of sugar and 3 g of fiber. That's wonderful!

If you grab a bunch of oranges, like 3 or 4 of them, and squeeze them to make juice, you get about 1 c of orange juice. You'd be getting 112 calories, including 21 g of sugar and *no fiber*. You get nearly *double* the calories and the sugar and no fiber to slow down its path to your bloodstream.

Now, I LOVE oranges and I have them on a regular basis. There was one time when I had gone to a workout on an empty stomach first thing in the morning, and then I went right to running errands and appointments and I didn't make it home for quite some time. I got hungry around 10:30 or 11, so I ate an orange. After that, I didn't get hungry again until at least noon. One orange sustained me for an hour or two, easily, even post-workout.

But what about 8 oz of orange juice? First of all, unless you were really watching carefully, you'd likely go back for a second glass, or you'd seek some other snack to fill you up.

Why is that? Even though it has *double* the calories and the sugar, the juice will never fill you up. The fiber is missing from the juice, and it's the fiber that is necessary to create bulk and to stimulate the feeling of fullness.

There's another important issue with fiber - it slows down digestion. That's a good thing! Not only does it keep you full longer, but the nutrients (including sugar) are introduced to the bloodstream much more slowly.

This is how a perfectly good food turns into a detrimental food. Even in something as simple as fresh-squeezed orange juice, that level of processing has a dramatic effect on weight gain and metabolism. This is not to scare you away from fruit juices altogether. If you're currently drinking soda pop then certainly orange juice is a better option. However, it would be good to work toward drinking most of your liquid as water as soon as you can manage. This will cut down on a great number of hidden calories and eating whole fruit instead of fruit juice will offer your body the perfect package of nutrients and fiber to keep your body nourished and feeling full.

To sum it up, when I recommend eating a whole food plant-based diet, I'm suggesting eating plants just about the same way they're found in nature. This is by far the most effective and safest way to lose weight because you'll be satiated and full without overeating calories. It's also the most effective way to optimize your health. You'll get to experience the health benefits of the micronutrients along with the satiety benefit of the fiber and water. When you eat food in the whole package that nature intended, the naturally occurring sugars are released so slowly into the bloodstream that you avoid the blood sugar spike, insulin rise, and the crash that usually follows.

Speaking of "crash" you just got a "crash course" in whole food plant-based nutrition!

So just remember, when you're confused about whether something qualifies as whole-food, ask this one question: Does it look like it did when it was growing or harvested???

If YES, carry on!

If Only Pasta Grew on Trees

CLIENT SPOTLIGHT
MEET SHARI

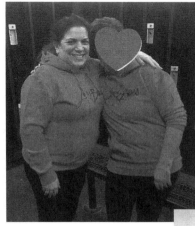

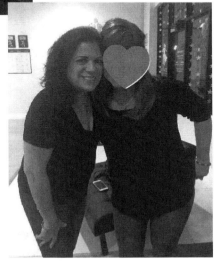

In 2017 I was following a weight loss plan that was not vegan and I couldn't figure out how to make it work for me. I was really frustrated by how long I'd been struggling with excess weight that wouldn't budge. When Christin broke it down the way she does, it finally made sense to me. Having that deeper understanding helped me to get back on track. I love the way the program is organized so that I could walk through it step by step. It addresses the emotional component of our behavior and addresses the whole person and not just the food. I love that it's not all about weight loss, but it's addressing optimal health which results in weight loss.

After working through the program, I finally understood *how* to be a WFPB eater. Prior to that, I thought I knew what to do but I just wasn't doing it. Now I understand exactly what was missing and how to keep it going.

It's so great for me to see my changes inspiring my teenage kids too. My ex-husband is vegan for medical reasons, so our houses are both clean of meat and dairy, and my kids are happily eating vegan even though they weren't raised that way.

I used to think that going out to eat was a huge treat, but then I realized that I was actually sabotaging myself with a lot of restaurant meals and some other snacks. In hindsight, it was the basics, not the complicated tricks, that really made a difference for me. And as much as I thought I could learn my way out of it on my own, I really needed the guidance of this program to pull it all together.

I am *not* a black and white person, and it was just too hard for me to try to stay compliant in the past. If I have to pick one thing, for me it was working on my daily PLANTS Targets to create balance instead of obsessing about my food.

Once I decided that all of my food must come from the Green Light area (at least for now), I saw crazy results! I finally experienced that calm brain that I'd heard so many people talk about. My moods are more stable. My mind is clear, and I feel more positive and optimistic. It's like the dark cloud that hung around me has finally lifted and I can see the light (and feel light!) for the first time in decades!

Now if I get off track, I *always* get right back on, and quickly! No more spiraling downhill for weeks or months at a time like I used to. I've gone on to all of the Forever Diet coaching programs and I've learned something new every time. It's as if my level of growth and development is infinite because I keep reaching new levels I didn't even know I was striving for!

> *I truly thought I was doing all the right things for so long, but I was still not seeing the results I wanted. When I began eating exclusively in the Green Light area, everything came together for me! I had no idea what an impact "a little bit here and there" was having on me. It was taking over my ability to make good decisions and it was dampening my mood. I'm so happy to be on the other side of that now, and I can't wait to see you cross that bridge too! You got this!*
>
> ~SHARI

READY, SET, ACTION! NOW IT'S YOUR TURN!

How are things going so far? Now that you have a new understanding of what really qualifies as a whole food, what are some things that have snuck into your diet, with or without your knowledge, that don't qualify as a whole food?

_____

_____

_____

_____

_____

_____

In what ways do you hope to see improvements from making the switch to more whole foods and fewer processed foods?

_____

_____

_____

_____

_____

_____

_____

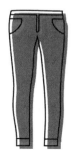

CHAPTER 8

Making Your Life Interesting with P.L.A.N.T.S.

Make your food boring and your life interesting.

~ ANDREW TAYLOR OF SPUD FIT

Oftentimes when people hear about a whole food plant-based diet, they start to wonder "Where do you get your protein?!" but instead, I think we should all be asking, "Where do you get your happiness?!"

It is common in our culture to use food to celebrate, to medicate, to grieve, to comfort, to cover up loneliness, depression, or anxiety.

For most of us, this starts in childhood. Happy memories are often anchored with some kind of sweet treat. This goes on for many years. And then later in life when we want to feel good, we subconsciously reach for sweet treats. We grab a calorie-dense "treat," get a rush of dopamine, and as a result, we temporarily feel good. This encourages us to repeat the behavior over and over again.

The problem is, we have stressors every single day pushing us to reach for those sweet treats, and they are *so* accessible. It's just plain easy to get your hands on something and shove it in your mouth!

If your childhood wasn't filled with happy memories, you may have taken a slightly different path to end up at the same place. Many times, children who are struggling at home will use food as a coping mechanism. Eating is one thing they feel like they can control, and so they eat to excess. Or they sneak food to get attention. There are all sorts of ways it can happen, but one way or another, most adults who are overweight have a history of using food to cope with something.

You deserve to get better and to feel better. Regardless of how you got here, you are not broken. We can simply take stock of where we are now. We can light the path forward for each other, and start moving. We got this, okay?

When work is stressful, we wander by the snacks in the break room and dig in. When home life is stressful, we wander to the kitchen. When we're stressed out by traffic, we're more prone to stopping at a gas station, fast food joint, coffee shop, or a restaurant to grab a quick dopamine-jolting 'pick-me-up'.

Dopamine from food is so readily available that it's all too common for this to eventually become our greatest source of feel-good hormones. And when food becomes your greatest source of "feel-good" hormones, look out. That is a recipe for disaster.

I'd like to share with you a quote that I just love by my friend Andrew SpudFit Taylor:

"Make your food boring and your LIFE interesting."

It's not that your food has to be boring at all. In fact, I enjoy my food more than I ever did previously! The point here is that your life must be interesting! If it's not, then you'll turn to food to meet your needs, and that spells trouble. This is precisely why I'm so strict about having fun! It's for your own good - literally!

So how else can we get a good dose of feel-good hormones??

If you have lived for many years relying on food for comfort, entertainment, joy, and friendship, then you must replace the food with other joys. If you just take away your main source of happiness (eg. animal products or processed food) without replacing it with something else, you won't have a sustainable future on your healthy eating plan. Your brain will seek dopamine or other happy hormones any way it can. And it will win.

Yep, that's right. Your brain's survival mechanism will win every time. In order to outsmart it, you've got to proactively set yourself up for success. It's your job to create other ways to make your life interesting that have nothing to do with food! Make your life more interesting and you won't need to rely on food for fun. Make sense?

Here are some other fun facts. Choosing plants over animals (especially choosing beans over meat) naturally increases the dopamine release in your brain.

Taking a brisk walk or other types of exercise for at least 20 minutes will increase your endorphins.

Living in gratitude will help increase your serotonin.

Developing quality relationships and giving to others actually increases oxytocin.

You know, it might be a good idea to remind yourself of these things every day, and even give yourself a checkmark when you do them! OOOOOOHHHH!!! I have an idea! You could even use the system I created, and start tracking your *PLANTS Targets* every day!!!

Let me explain. The PLANTS acronym is a system I've created to help you focus on doing the right things, just a little bit each day, to really help you move the needle quickly. Throughout the day, you'll check off your targets as you earn them, and by the end of the day, you'll see how many you've earned.

Here's what each letter of the acronym means:

P is for Planning Ahead to make sure you have your healthy food at the ready. You'll want to get in the habit of preparing food in advance. You may wish to do a big food prep day once a week or you may prefer to do a few smaller prep days throughout the week. Anticipating challenges like going to your friends' house or a restaurant will go a long way in keeping you on track. Think ahead about what you'll do when you go outside of your safety bubble so you don't get goo-goo in front of temptation and kick yourself later. If you're anticipating challenges in your day and Planning Ahead, you earn your P. Simple as that. Check it off!

L is for LOTS of Healthy Food from the Green Light area which will help you feel full, and it'll have a positive effect on your happy hormones. My ultimate suggestion is that you eat exclusively WFPB (whole-food plant-based) which means you're eating exclusively from the Green Light area and only having a little bit of Yellow Light foods if that's part of your plan at this time. Each person's food plan will vary slightly, so this target is open to your own interpretation. I'll just ask you to be clear *with yourself* about your own rules and plans. In other words, you're free to draw the line in the sand wherever you want, and you can adjust it as you go, but don't forget to draw the line.

Let's say you're brand new and this is the first time you're moving away from animal products and processed foods. For the first couple of weeks, you might earn your L as long as you incorporate a big salad at some point during the day. And after that, you might get your L as long as you stay away from dairy. After that, as long as you stay away from meat and dairy. And after that, as long as you stay in the Green Light and Yellow Light areas.

If you've been at this a while, you may make the plan to eat all of your food from the Green Light area for the next 30 days, so you only earn your L if you stick with that plan. If you're somewhere in the middle, maybe you eat from the Green Light area plus some tofu and tempeh. There's no right or wrong here. Your schedule is your own, and there's no wrong way to succeed. The important thing is to be intentional about moving along a spectrum toward the Green Light area and to eventually include some healthy foods from the Yellow Light area as long as they're not problematic for you.

The P and the L represent the food portion of the program. The other 4 targets are for everything else. Remember when I said that this is not a diet? It's not all about the food! As evidence, four of the six daily targets have nothing to do with food!

A is for Activity which boosts your happy hormones, so if you do at least a little bit every day, you'll earn your A. Bear in mind, this doesn't have to be 90 minutes at the gym 6 days a week! This can be parking at the far side of the parking lot, taking the stairs instead of the elevator, or even walking the dog. Another great strategy is to do squats or stretches in front of the TV during commercials rather than sitting on the couch! If you've made some intentional activity part of your day, you earn your A.

N is for Nice, as in being a nice person! Here's where it gets really fun. You see, being a nice person means you're building relationships and boosting your oxytocin. Having your happy hormones flowing is going to make sticking with this program a whole lot easier. It's what makes this program different from other things out there. Being a nice person is part of your homework, every day. Pay someone a compliment, offer a random act of kindness, and BOOM! There's your check for N! I told you I was going to make this easy.

T is for being Thankful and living in gratitude, which boosts your serotonin and your overall mood. Many studies have shown the positive effects that take place when we are focusing on gratitude instead of lack. Life becomes easier almost instantly when you can shift your thoughts to a place of genuine gratitude. Incorporate this practice into your life, and you'll never be the same. Think of a few things you're truly thankful for, and you've earned your T for the day.

S is for Sleep. Making sure you get enough sleep is important for your happy hormones and all bodily functions. When you get enough sleep, you're pumping the brakes on your overscheduled, stressful life. You're shutting down your fight or flight response and you're turning on your rest and digest system. This allows your body to heal from the inside out. Get your 8-9 hours of sleep each night and you've earned your S for sleep.

The best way to use this system is to watch for trends over time. Every day for 7 days, track your PLANTS Targets.

Make it a game and see how many letters you can earn. At the end of 7 days, count them all up and divide by 42 which is the maximum number of targets.

Remember, we're not looking for 100%. We're looking for hitting 80% of your targets, on average, over the course of a week. Keep an eye on this and I guarantee that you'll see a predictable trend. The closer your targets are to 80%, the faster you'll get back in your pants!

The beauty of this system is that it is so simple. It focuses on what is most important without overcomplicating things. If you use the PLANTS Targets acronym as a daily reminder of the most important things to focus on and tally them up at the end of the week to evaluate and make adjustments, then you're going to succeed. There can be no other way.

PLANTS Targets are the key to finding balance, making your life interesting, and making sure you stay on the fast track to success.

Making Your Life Interestingwith P.L.A.N.T.S.

CLIENT SPOTLIGHT
MEET NIKKI

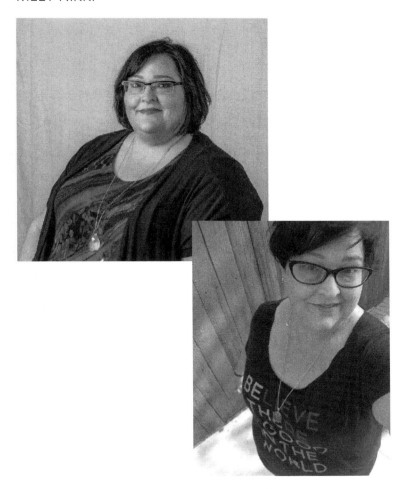

When I started on my journey to have a healthful life, my first plan was to have gastric bypass surgery. I had lost the same 100 pounds over and over again and could never find a way to make it last or to get lower than that. I thank my lucky stars that I found WFPB eating in time and realized I didn't need bypass surgery. I got started by following Dr. Greger and Forks Over Knives and some other plant-based programs. They helped, but I needed to go to a deeper level to really get a handle on it. I had lost 75 lbs or more but started going back to old habits. Being able to buy cute clothes and take flattering pictures just was not enough to keep me on track!

Along the way, I realized that the problem was far deeper than just the physical things you can see on the outside. I'm diabetic and suffer from bipolar disorder. I was a victim of severe trauma and I went through a challenging year of EMDR therapy. The support that I got from Christin and TransformU aligned with my other work, and healing the deeper stuff has totally changed the way I feel about my issues with food addiction.

The excess weight was just a symptom, and if I had tried to fix it with surgery, it would have just kept coming back. Going a little deeper and recognizing what was really going on kept me on the path. My appearance on the outside was just a byproduct of my decisions which were driven by mental and emotional factors. That wasn't going to change until I really got to the root of the problem and dealt with it.

This program lined up with all the other things I was doing for myself, and the holistic approach was exactly what I needed. Gaining and losing weight had always been a struggle in the past. I can't even believe I get to say this, but I have now overcome that vicious cycle. I'm on a much more stable path, and I've learned how to see what's really going on so I address it head-on.

For example, I used to really go down a spiral of negative thinking and self-hatred when I went off-plan. It fueled my thoughts of being a bad person, of not doing well, and then I would go further off and not come back.

Now I can have a bad moment and the next thing I put in my mouth can get me right back on track. It doesn't have to derail me like it used to. If you look around elsewhere on social media, it looks like everyone else is doing just perfectly, but they're not! It's important to remember that it's working, and this is the right path, even if the process is sometimes slower.

During quarantine, I needed to stay closer to the group because I got overwhelmed and my schedule completely changed. I also got private coaching from Christin to help me get a routine in place which kept me from getting overwhelmed, and that helped me stick with my plan.

I move my body every day, not to burn calories but to keep my head on straight! I find a way to have fun and do things that make me laugh. I started a veggie garden and I connect with people that I care about. All of these things are consistent with the PLANTS targets, and this holistic approach to my life has made all of the difference this time.

In reality, the path through life is full of bumps and curves, and having the support of this program gave me the tools I need to handle those bumps rather than continuing to get thrown off by them.

It has given me control of my life back.

> *It makes such a difference to have an objective way to view progress, not only to keep myself honest but to make sure I recognize all the things I'm doing right. Left to my own devices, I would do a pretty decent job, but if I missed one thing, I'd really beat myself up and chalk up the day as a failure. Thanks to the PLANTS system, I don't do that anymore. It forces me to recognize what I'm doing right and it's a constant reminder that every little bit counts! Even being nice to strangers on the street gets me an N for Nice, and it's moving me closer to my goals. Don't put it off.*
> *Start today!*
>
> ~NIKKI

READY, SET, ACTION! NOW IT'S YOUR TURN!

It's time to start tracking your own PLANTS targets. Consider what your rules will be for each one, and then start tracking! Use this chart to track your next 7 days, and then tally up the total at the end of the week. Don't wait until Sunday or Monday to start. Do it today and you'll feel so glad that you did! Continue for the next few weeks in this book, and then download and print your own copies from www.theforeverdiet.org/book-bonuses.

Plants TARGETS TRACKER

P = Plan Ahead L = Lots of Healthy Food A = Actiivty N = Nice T = Thankful S = Sleep

For each day, put a checkmark for each target that you earn. Track daily, and at the end of each 7 days, we'll tally up the totals. We're shooting for hitting 80% of our PLANTS targets on average each week. Use this simple feedback to keep yourself accountable.

	Date	P	L	A	N	T	S	#
Ex.	6/1	✓	✓		✓	✓		4
1								
2				**EXAMPLE**				
3								
4			**Use the Plants Target Trackers on the next few**					
5			**pages to track your daily progress.**					
6								
7								
						Total # this week		
						Total # ÷ 42 x 100 =		%

How do you feel? Note any connections as time goes on!

Plants
TARGETS TRACKER

	Date	P	L	A	N	T	S	#
Ex:	6/1	✓	✓		✓	✓		4
1								
2								
3								
4								
5								
6								
7								

Total # this week

Total # ÷ 42 × 100 = ____ %

How do you feel? Note any connections as time goes on!

Plants
TARGETS TRACKER

Date	P	L	A	N	T	S	#
Ex: 6/1	✓	✓		✓	✓		4
1							
2							
3							
4							
5							
6							
7							

Total # this week

Total # ÷ 42 × 100 = _____ %

How do you feel? Note any connections as time goes on!

Plants TARGETS TRACKER

Date	P	L	A	N	T	S	#
Ex: 6/1	✓	✓		✓	✓		4
1							
2							
3							
4							
5							
6							
7							

Total # this week

Total # ÷ 42 × 100 = _____ %

How do you feel? Note any connections as time goes on!

_____

_____

Plants
TARGETS TRACKER

	Date	P	L	A	N	T	S	#
Ex:	6/1	✓	✓		✓	✓		4
1								
2								
3								
4								
5								
6								
7								

Total # this week

Total # ÷ 42 x 100 = _____ %

How do you feel? Note any connections as time goes on!

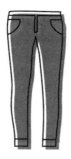

CHAPTER 9

A for Activity

Sweat is magic. Cover yourself in it daily to grant your wishes.

~UNKNOWN

First things first, let's do a little vocabulary check, shall we? There's a reason I use A for Activity instead of E for exercise. Here's the deal. We're not just trying to get you to go out and get a new gym membership or join a cardio or weight lifting class, show up for 45-60 minutes, check it off your list, and then go sit in your desk chair all day. That's actually not the objective at all. You see, the benefits of exercise are cumulative, and the setbacks from being sedentary are cumulative as well.

So yes, it's wonderful if you're already in the habit of going to the gym or exercising regularly throughout the week. Keep doing it! Let's say you're exercising for one hour. What are you doing for the other 23 hours a day? Sleeping for lots of it, I hope, but then you're sitting in your car, sitting at a desk to work, sitting at the table to eat, sitting on the couch to relax. If you had a stopwatch that started every time you sat down or laid down and stopped every time you got up, I bet you'd be shocked at how many hours every day you spend in a sedentary position.

Some of this is unavoidable, I know! Standing toilets are not coming any time soon. Self-driving cars, yes, but I doubt the gas pedal is about to be turned into a recumbent bike. Actually, that's brilliant, isn't it?! Wanna go faster? Better pedal faster!

That said, there are some workarounds! Let's say you work at a desk most of the time. The best thing you can do is get up from your chair, walk around, move around, and get some kind of activity in for some period of time! No, you don't have to go run up and down 5 flights of stairs between phone calls, unless of course, you want to. But you do want to find a way to get some activity in.

Let's say you get up and you do a simple box step in your cubicle. This is a great mental exercise too. Start with your feet together, in the bottom left corner of an imaginary box. Then with your left foot, step forward to the top left corner of the box, then slide your right foot to the top right corner. Bring your left foot over to meet the right. Step back to the bottom right corner with your right foot, then slide your left foot to the bottom left corner. Bring your feet together, back to where you started. Go slowly to start.

Hang on to something if you need to. Make sure you don't fall over.

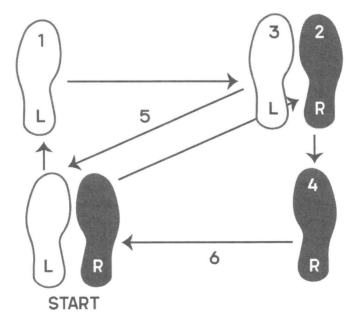

Once you get the hang of it, could you manage to do that if you were on a conference call? Probably, right? Could you pick up the speed? Could you add some upper body movements too? Tell me this is too easy for you and I'll show you how to do this with dumbbells or even my favorite - box step burpees! There's always a way to up the intensity; don't worry about that, my friend.!

Retrain yourself to sneak in little bits of activity throughout the day. The best way I know to actually *do* this is to set an alarm on your phone. You can set it to go off every hour as a reminder to get some activity in. I'll even give you a checklist of ideas so that you always have something at the top of your mind to do! You could post it in your kitchen, and while you're waiting for something in the microwave, the oven, or the Instant Pot, work on one or two of the items on your list! Pop into www.theForeverDiet.org/Book-Bonuses for the checklist.

The idea is to create ways to get activity into your existing routine. There's another reason why I highly recommend this method. If you define exercise as a 45-60 minute event, then you either do it or you don't. There's no partial credit. So you either feel great, or you may feel like a bum. Or, you may feel so totally overwhelmed at the thought of even trying to carve an extra 45-60 minutes out of the day for a home workout, plus a commute to a gym and back, and there's just no way it's going to happen.

Let's say you commit to doing it because you're fed up and need to get into shape. So now you're going 4-5 days a week, and things are going great!

Until... life pops up again and you can't make it.

And now you're back to doing nothing. You'd gotten used to getting all those happy hormones from your once-a-day workout, and you get cut off. Uh oh.

What if there was a better way? What if rather than one single workout, you broke it down into micro-activities throughout the day? You get out of bed in the morning, and before you hop in the shower you do a few gentle knee raises or march in place. While you're brushing your teeth you're standing on one foot. Now you're working on balance and some fine stabilizing muscles that don't get worked very often! Hold on to the counter at first so you don't fall over, please!

Whenever you leave the house, you park kinda far away from the door. You take the stairs instead of the elevator whenever possible. Throughout the day you can sit on a stability ball to build core strength, you can do a few movements with dumbbells or exercise bands, and every hour you've got a little alarm going off reminding you to get up and do something! Just for 2 minutes.

That's 7-8 times just during your workday that you're getting up and doing some kind of activity. You get home, and maybe while dinner is cooking, you do some wall push-ups or counter push-ups. Maybe you do some dips on a kitchen chair. If you do sit down to watch tv, get up during the commercials and get some more activity in. Work your way through that checklist each day and see how many of the activities you can check off.

Do you know how much time that method will cost you? *Maybe* 15 minutes extra, mainly for parking farther away, taking the stairs, etc. And what did you do? You got in a 30-45 minute "workout" in little spurts all throughout the day!

Studies have shown that little bursts of activity are as effective or more effective than one sustained period of activity once a day. And you know what's most important about that? Even on a bad day, you're still always doing something! It's working within the shades of gray, not the black and white, where you will find the greatest success.

If you do this consistently, it can easily become part of your regular routine. It's never daunting to get started, and you'll take action, which will inspire you to take more action. When you do that, you're always more likely to find success. That makes you feel good, and that is going to make you more likely to do it again tomorrow!

This is really starting to sound like the path to success, and you're on it.

A for Activity

CLIENT SPOTLIGHT
MEET VICKY

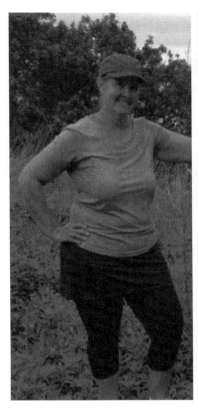
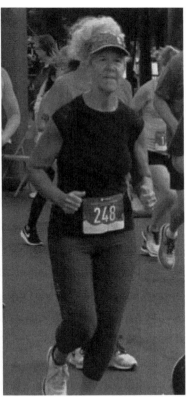

My mom had surgery - two heart attacks and open-heart surgery, and she was never the same again. Her five girls were all overweight, and I knew I had to do something. The thought of my own kids gathered around my hospital bed waiting to see if I'd survive was just too hard for me to bear.

I made many attempts at weight loss over the years, but when I found out I had Rheumatoid Arthritis, it started my search for cleaner plant-based solutions. I lost a lot of weight and realized I could finally keep it off quite easily. Unfortunately, early in my journey, everything else I'd tried was unsustainable. I was so discouraged that I couldn't do it. I was tempted to just throw in the towel.

I'm so thankful that I found Christin's programs because I finally understood it wasn't just about the food. It was the system and the methodology behind it.

Having the mindset tools from Christin's programs made all the difference for me. I love the positive aspect of Christin's program. The support that's available is amazing too. I have a wonderful loving husband who supports me in my efforts, but he has no interest in eating like I do. It's been a challenge since we're together so much and we travel many months of the year in an RV. We're always going to new restaurants and coming across new situations that I have to navigate, but since I've done the mindset training, this has become a way of life for me, and it's no longer challenging.

I'm not perfect, don't get me wrong, but I sure do feel like I have it all together, which is something I never thought I'd say. After seeing my outcomes, three of my sisters have started eating more vegan. They have lost a significant amount of weight and it's so rewarding to see them inspired by my changes

This program has totally improved the way I relate to other people who don't eat like me! I used to judge other people or feel compelled to save them or impose my help upon them. Now I just inspire them without even trying! Christin's way of helping with my mindset has made all of the difference. I'm more confident than I've ever been, and I've been able to navigate some really challenging situations that would have sent the old me into a downward spiral that might have lasted months.

The Facebook group is just so supportive and helpful, and it's such a joy to have met so many like-minded people on this journey that I now call friends. I only wish I'd found this sooner! It would have saved me a lot of heartache and frustration!

I can't even tell you what a difference it made when I started sneaking in activity. When I viewed it as a gift for my body and a boost for my mood, I really prioritized making it happen. It became less about burning calories and more about a celebration for what my body could do! It encouraged me to keep testing my limits in a positive way!

~VICKY

READY, SET, ACTION! NOW IT'S YOUR TURN!

It's all too common to think we don't have enough time in the day to fit in one more thing. So let's start by using your time more wisely. Where in your day can you sneak in some activity rather than being idle?

_____
_____
_____
_____
_____
_____
_____
_____
_____
_____

For the next 7 days, see if you can get in at least one session of additional activity, even 5 minutes, that you wouldn't have otherwise. How about starting right now?

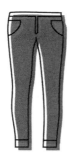

CHAPTER 10

It Takes a Village

Alone we can do so little. Together we can do so much.
~HELEN KELLER

Each year the whole food plant-based lifestyle gets more and more mainstream, but let's face it, it's going to be a while before health and happiness are consistently prioritized over profits. The temptations of junk food far outweigh the quiet call of the humble vegetable, and it's something we'll always want to be conscious about.

Food manufacturers know this quite well. If they want to sell you something, they'll douse it in artificially high amounts of salt, oil, and sugar in order to zap your tastebuds. This also sets your pleasure centers on fire, and before you know it, you really can't eat just one, no matter how determined you are, and no matter how much you "know."

Food advertisers know that exposure and repetition are too much for most of us to overcome. It's no accident that we find candy bars at the gas station, snack vending machines at the library, double bacon cheeseburgers on a bus stop advertisement, and billboards loaded with milkshakes and fries. We see chips in the check-out line at the hardware store and a candy dish in every waiting room. Coffee beverages have become a full day's worth of calories, and they look as enticing as an ice cream sundae.

Heck. My mouth is watering even writing this because I can see the images in my head. That's how powerfully conditioned we have become. I haven't eaten most of those things in years; I have no desire for a cheeseburger, and yet…

I'm literally salivating at the image. Wow.

The reality is, we live in an environment that is full of temptations. It is not designed for wellness or weight loss.

Instead, the real world we live in is designed to sell us food (and drugs) that will keep us fat and sick and miserable. If we proceed down this path, we'll eventually be so miserable we have no choice but to drown our sorrows in more junk food, and we'll turn to more prescription drugs to fix our growing list of ailments.

Unless... we choose a different path.

If we choose a path of unconditional love for ourselves and others, then we'll see things differently. We will see food as fuel that keeps our bodies running in optimum condition. We will choose health-promoting foods and we'll feel excited about it. We'll realize that deprivation comes from a life of disability, not a life without junk food.

We will finally see a different result and we will create a different life.

In a world where it's increasingly normal to drop dead of a heart attack in your 60s, I'll take a pass on normal, thank you very much.

It can be hard to stand out though. It can be hard to make choices that are counter to the mainstream. It can feel like an uphill battle and some days can be discouraging. I've told you before, and I'll tell you again something that you can always fall back on:

You are never alone on this journey.

If you look around, you'll see so many others who are waking up to a better future. We are filled with hope, optimism, and confidence. We are ready to help a friend in need because we realize that we did not arrive here alone, and you needn't do it alone either.

It truly takes a village to find success, and I've made it

my mission is to offer you a village full of supporters, cheerleaders, and champions. I have compiled my most impactful training into an online coaching program so that we can work together in the comfort of your own home. M365 offers the motivation to keep you moving forward, one day at a time and it's the seat belt that keeps you on the ride even when life throws you for a loop. By going far beyond the food and getting to the root of the problems that are actually keeping you from progress, you'll be able to sustain amazing successes.

The folks in my program are the most supportive, genuine and engaging people I have had the pleasure of knowing, and we're all ready to cheer you on next.

Every day I see raw vulnerable struggle followed by a rush of support. I see Voyagers sharing their experience and compassion.

We call ourselves Voyagers because a voyage is defined as "a long journey." The journey to wellness is a long journey. Sometimes it takes awhile to get there but even if we arrive quickly it's important to stay there long-term.

I see stories of triumph and a genuine delight from the crowd. There is no competition among us, and in fact we all rise a little higher and our hope burns even brighter when each person shares a win. There's a gentle drive for today's version of myself to be a little bit better than yesterday's.

I'm right there too, offering support, encouragement, and a gentle nudge to keep you moving forward. If you've been resonating with my philosophy, my methods, and the tools in this book, then you'll love taking this next step in your journey together.

It is my greatest wish that each person can have the opportunity in this lifetime to realize their true value. I hope that you can someday see what it is that I already see in you - a person who is worthy of love and worthy of a healthy happy life.

When you can shift to see things this way, then living a healthy and happy lifestyle will not only be feasible for you, but undeniable. This, my friend, is the key to everlasting success, which also happens to be my greatest wish for you.

Baby Got Back in Her Pants

CLIENT SPOTLIGHT
MEET JANICE

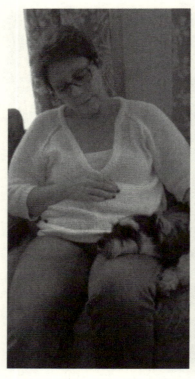
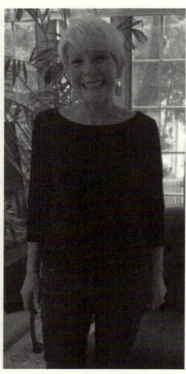

I have really struggled with my weight for most of my adult life and while I knew that eating plant-based was the healthiest way for me to live, I was really having trouble sticking with it. I have tried so many different programs over the years, investing thousands of dollars in the process, and I had little to show for it.

I'm a shy person, and it was hard for me to open up in other support groups. But since I've started working more closely with Christin, it's been such a breath of fresh air! She doesn't chastise you for anything. In fact, when I make a bad decision, she's the first to remind me that I'm not bad and that it's perfectly normal to not be perfect.

I shifted my focus from weight loss to long-term health, and I dug deep to understand my true motivations. Tapping in to what drives my decisions has helped to guide me ever since.

Even in the midst of the COVID-19 pandemic, I was on top of my game. I'm walking every single day, I'm meditating, and I'm preparing healthy food. I've fallen in love with playing the piano all over again, a pleasure I had denied myself for too long. My clothes are looser than ever, and I'm feeling more positive and hopeful than ever before.

I am so grateful to be armed with a skill set that is helping me to succeed despite any circumstances on the outside. I have embraced a well-balanced life by taking one day at a time, and it has made all the difference.

The Forever Diet coaching programs really motivated me to do my best. I final-ly realized that I am worthy of good health, and I have learned that it's about so much more than just the food. After decades of dieting, I was so focused on the food. I was hyper-aware of everything I ate and I beat myself up for every bite that was off-plan. It took me a while to let go of that, but I finally have. I hope that you'll follow your heart and join me as a Voyager so I can cheer for you as so many others have cheered for me!

~JANICE

READY, SET, ACTION! NOW IT'S YOUR TURN!

The journey to healthy living is lined with so many gifts. There is hope, happiness, and joy all along the way if you choose to embrace it. You've got the knowledge, you've started to implement, and now it's time to make sure you never go back to where you started.

You can succeed, and you deserve to succeed. The road ahead comes with its twists and turns, and plenty of surprises. There will be new times of stress, and times where you're not sure you can continue. It is imperative that you have the support you need when those times arise.

Life is like a roller coaster with its ups and downs, and thank goodness! How boring would it be otherwise? Life can throw you for a loop, and as long as you've got your safety belt on, you'll be able to stay on the ride of your life no matter what. It will keep you moving toward success even if no one else is supportive, even if you travel frequently, even if you have a terrible family history, and even if you have no willpower whatsoever.

I created a program called M365 where you can have daily contact, live interactions, and powerfully concise nuggets of motivation to spur you forward in your quest for health and happiness. We never expect anyone to be perfect, and this is your best opportunity to navigate the path forward with all of the support, love and encouragement it takes to truly thrive.

Join us now at

www.theforeverdiet.org/motivation

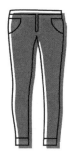

RECIPES

Baby Got Back in Her Pants

AIR-FRIED ONION RINGS

Everyone's looking for a crunchy snack. And have I got the answer for you?! I've perfected the method for crispy, delicious onion rings, and you'll just have to try it for yourself to see if you agree!

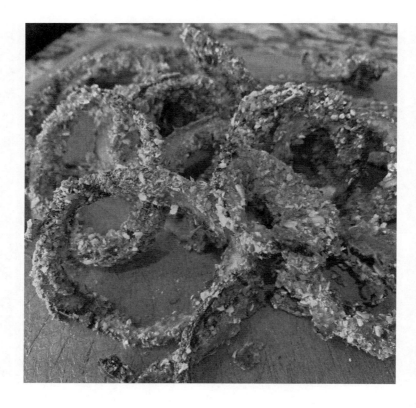

PREP TIME: 5 Minutes

COOK TIME: 14 Minutes

YIELD: 3 Servings

INGREDIENTS:

1 Large sweet onion (Vidalias or Mayan Sweets work great), sliced and separated into rings.

3 Tbsp aquafaba (liquid from cooked or canned beans)

2 Tbs water

COATING:

1/2 c ground oats

1/3 c nutritional yeast

3 Tbsp ground flax

1 Tbsp Italian seasoning

2 tsp onion powder

1 tsp black pepper

INSTRUCTIONS:

Combine aquafaba and water.

Dip the onion rings in aquafaba + water, and then place in shallowpan with coating.

Flip to coat both sides.

Lay in a single layer in air fryer.

Cook at 390 degrees for 12-14 minutes, checking periodically.

Let cool slightly before enjoying!

BANANA BREAD OVERNIGHT OATS

Make a batch or two of this oatmeal and you'll have a "home-cooked" breakfast ready to grab and go! No more babysitting oats over the stovetop and reheating a gummy mess the next day. This will easily maintain its texture and delicious flavor!

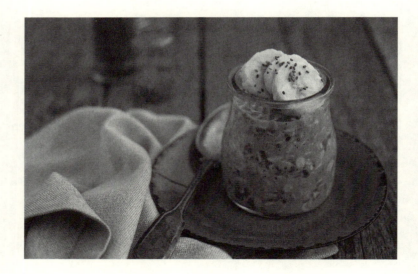

PREP TIME: 2 Minutes

REFRIGERATE: Overnight

YIELD: 4 Servings

INGREDIENTS:

2 c rolled oats

2 bananas, mashed

2 c non-dairy milk

2 Tbsp chia seeds or ground flax seeds *(optional)*

2 tsp cinnamon

1 tsp cardamom

INSTRUCTIONS:

Add all ingredients to a mixing bowl, combine.

Store in refrigerator overnight.

Stir and serve warm or cold.

Serve plain or top with fresh berries.

If oats aren't your thing, you can try this recipe with cooked rice or quinoa to mix it up. Reduce milk by ½ cup.

CHERRY BERRY INSTANT RICE PUDDING

Having started my plant-based journey because of a high blood pressure scare, I was particularly pleased to learn how beets can help your blood vessels dilate and stay nice and stretchy. Anthocyanins, found in tart cherries, are well known to help with inflammation and speed recovery. Beet Boost just happens to be a combination of both! Add that to the fact that they just released a new cherry flavor, and whoa.... *swoon!

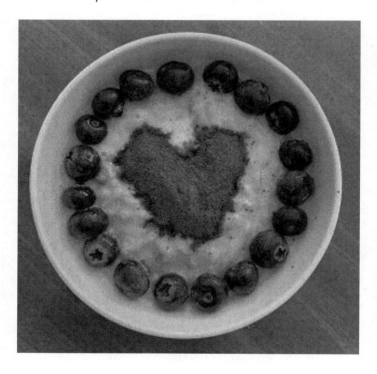

PREP TIME: 2 Minutes

COOK TIME: 1 Minute

YIELD: 1 Servings

INGREDIENTS:

1.5 cups cooked brown rice (I often make a rice/quinoa,/lentils blend, but anything works!)

1 ripe banana, mashed

1/4 – 1/3 cup unsweetened almond milk

1-2 Tbsp Cherry Beet Boost (new flavor!)

1/2 c blueberries

INSTRUCTIONS:

Mash banana, add milk and mash again to mix.

Stir in rain of choice.

Microwave 45 seconds and stir again.

Add more milk for desired consistency.

Top with Cherry Beet Boost and blueberries.

Serve and enjoy!

You can stir in the Beet Boost as you eat it, or you can take a little spoonful with each bite, however you fancy!

CHICKPEA SALAD

If I was stranded on a deserted island and could only take one food item with me, it would be chickpeas. Or maybe Japanese Sweet Potatoes. Or chickpeas… It's a toss-up. Either way, this fresh salad is composed of carrots, chickpeas, and avocado. It's tasty in all the right ways!

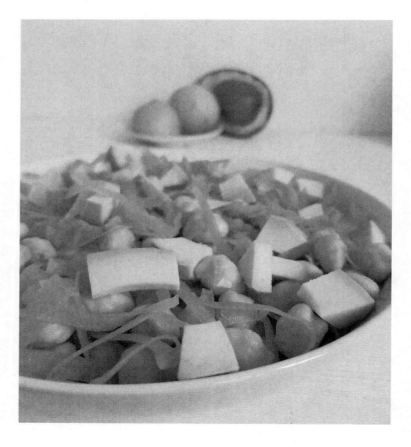

PREP TIME: 5 Minutes

COOK TIME: N/A

YIELD: 6 Servings

INGREDIENTS:

2 avocados, cubed

2 c chickpeas, cooked or canned, rinsed and drained

2 carrots, grated (or chopped if you prefer a crunch)

4 Tbsp lemon juice

1 tsp ground ginger

INSTRUCTIONS:

In a large bowl, combine lemon juice and ginger, mix well.

Add the chickpeas, avocados, and carrots.

Toss or stir gently until the ingredients are generously coated.

CHRISTIN'S POWER BREAKFAST

This is my favorite post-workout breakfast. It's packed with protein and heart healthy nutrients, with just enough sweetness to make it delicious.

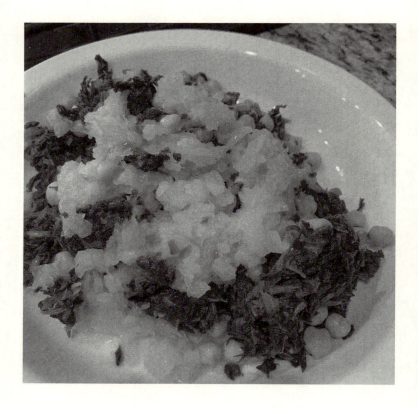

PREP TIME: 8 Minutes

COOK TIME: N/A

YIELD: 4 Servings

INGREDIENTS:

32 oz frozen chopped spinach

16 oz crushed pineapple in juice

3 c cooked chickpeas (30 oz canned)

½ - 1 Tbsp cinnamon

INSTRUCTIONS:

Thaw spinach in colander under hot water.

Squeeze excess water.

Drain and rinse chickpeas.

Transfer to mixing bowl.

Add pineapple and cinnamon and stir with a fork.

COOKIE DOUGH BALLS

You know how everyone loves to eat cookie dough, but when there are raw eggs it's really not the best idea? And even if the recipe is vegan, you'd feel a little naughty eating cookie dough, right? Well what if you could eat cookie dough that was made with beans and heart-healthy oats? Go ahead and eat your heart out!

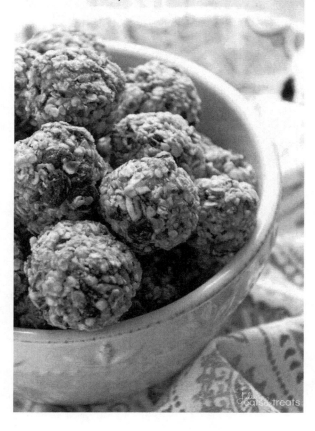

PREP TIME: 10 Minutes

COOK TIME: N/A

YIELD: 2 Dozen Balls

INGREDIENTS:

2 c rolled oats

1 c pitted dates

1 c cannellini beans, save water when you drain them!

1 tsp cinnamon

¼ tsp nutmeg

2 Tbsp aquafaba - the bean water you saved

1/4 cup dried currants or unsweetened non-dairy dark chocolate chunks *(optional)*

INSTRUCTIONS:

Place all ingredients except aquafaba and optional add-ins in food processor and blend until smooth.

Add the bean water as needed to achieve desired consistency.

Dough will start to form a ball on the blade.

Stir in optional add-ins.

Roll into 1 Tbsp balls and serve immediately or store in refrigerator.

Note: If they don't hold together well, add more liquid ½ Tbsp at a time until they do.

Baby Got Back in Her Pants

GREEN BEANS & KABOCHA SQUASH

This dish just screams fall. There is something magical about the combination of green beans and squash. The bright healthful colors look gorgeous together, and a drizzle of a nicely reduced balsamic vinegar turns this two ingredient dish into a crowd pleaser. Sometimes the simple taste is exactly what you need!

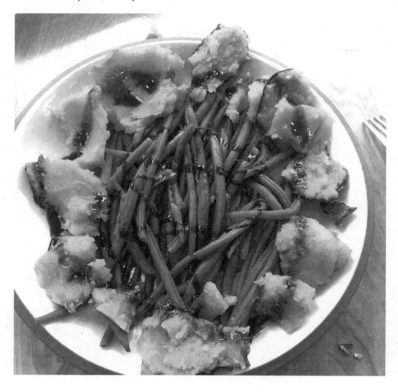

PREP TIME: 3 Minutes

COOK TIME: 20 Minute

YIELD: 4 Servings

INGREDIENTS:

2 lb green beans
1 large kabocha squash
balsamic vinegar

INSTRUCTIONS:

Put the whole kabocha on a steamer rack in the Instant Pot and cook for 7 minutes with 1 cup of water.

Quick release pressure.

While the squash is cooking, cook the beans in a large pot on the stovetop with cup of water.

Bring to a boil, lower heat to medium, cover and steam for 5-7 minutes to desired consistency.

When kabocha is complete, carefully remove from Instant Pot.

Cut in half and remove seeds and pulp.

Remove any bumps or scars on the squash's skin.

Leaving the rest of the skin intact, cut the squash into bite sized chunks.

Drain the green beans.

Cut into bite sized pieces if desired or serve whole.

Serve with squash on top and drizzle with a reduced balsamic vinegar such as Napa Valley Naturals Grand Reserve.

GUILT-FREE WAFFLES

This is my most-loved breakfast recipe from my blog. It turns a decadent splurge breakfast into something you can count as healthy and eat until you're totally stuffed without any guilt!

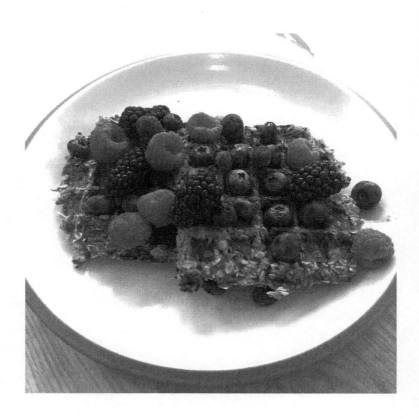

PREP TIME: 5 Minutes

COOK TIME: 20-25 Minutes

YIELD: 4 Classic Waffles

INGREDIENTS:

2 Tbsp ground flax seed

6 Tbsp warm water

2 ripe bananas, mashed

¼ c oat milk (soy and almond work great too)

1 ½ c fresh fruit, chopped. Raspberries, mango, strawberries, and blueberries make for a delightful treat but most fruit will work great.

1 tsp cinnamon

1/2 tsp vanilla

1 Tbsp chia seeds and hemp seeds *(optional)*

2 ½-3 c rolled oats

INSTRUCTIONS:

Preheat waffle iron.

Combine flax and water and set aside to thicken.

Combine bananas and milk first then add oats, cinnamon, vanilla, and optional seeds.

Stir in flax and water mixture which will act like an egg to bind ingredients better.

Spoon batter onto hot waffle iron, filling all the nooks and crannies.

Let run for the full cycle and then another 2-3 minutes.

Use a rubber spatula to peel the waffles off the iron.

Top with fresh fruit and a light sprinkle of cinnamon.

Baby Got Back in Her Pants

INSTANT POT VEGGIES AND STARCH

Sometimes we make cooking WAY harder than it needs to be. 75% of our meals in a week look something like this! It's nice to have the fun recipes, but it's also very freeing to keep it simple and realistic.

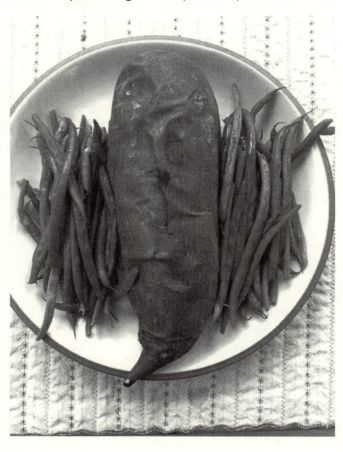

PREP TIME: 1 Minutes

COOK TIME: Varies

YIELD: Deliciousness

INGREDIENTS:

your favorite veggies
your favorite starches

INSTRUCTIONS:

Steam your favorite veggies, potatoes, and squash in the Instant Pot according to the following timetables. Add 1 cup of water and use the natural re leas e. Yo ur texture preferences may vary, but this is a general guide:

VEGGIES:

1 cup of water, QUICK release

Brussels Sprouts: 3 min (whole)

Green Beans: 1 min

Carrots: 1 min

Broccoli: 0 min

Cauliflower: 0 min

STARCHES:

1 cup of water, steamer rack, natural release

Potatoes *(cut into medium chunks)*: 4-5 mins

Potatoes (whole): 8-12 mins depending on size

Sweet Potatoes (whole): 10-15 mins depending on size

Acorn squash, whole: 7-8 minutes

Butternut squash, whole: 25 minutes

Kabocha squash, whole: 8-10 minutes

Spaghetti squash, whole; 6-8 minutes

JACKPOT (JACKFRUIT) CHILI

This recipe does have more ingredients than most of my other recipes, but since most of them are canned, or spices, the only thing you're actually chopping up are the onions and the jackfruit! It's actually a lot easier and faster to prepare than it might look at first glance.

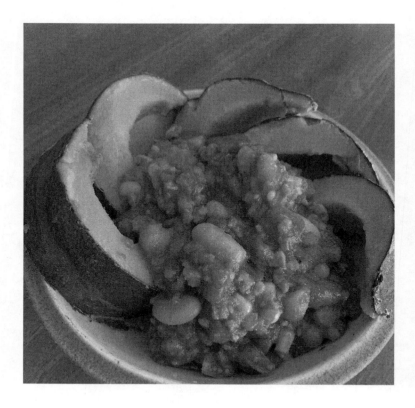

PREP TIME: 15 Minutes

COOK TIME: 35 Minutes

YIELD: 6-8 Servings

INGREDIENTS:

2 c onion, chopped (about 1 large)

1/4 c water

4 tsp dried oregano

1 tsp ground turmeric

1/4 tsp black pepper

1/2 tsp chili powder

1 4 oz can mild green chiles (medium for more kick)

1/2 c tomato paste

2 15 oz cans diced tomatoes (fire roasted for more kick)

2 15 oz cans kidney beans, drained and rinsed

2 15 oz cans pinto beans, drained and rinsed

1 15 oz can chickpeas, drained and rinsed

3 Tbsp Smoked Hickory Balsamic*

1 Tbsp Stone Ground Mustard

1 1/2 c mild salsa (medium for more kick)

4 halves canned pears, chopped

1 20 oz can jackfruit, chopped

INSTRUCTIONS:

Cook onions in water in a large pot over medium-high heat.

Cook until almost translucent, then add spices, green chiles, and tomato paste.

Cook 3-4 minutes, stirring frequently.

Add remaining ingredients.

Bring to a low boil.

Reduce heat and simmer 20-30 minutes.

*Chef's Note:
I highly recommend www.CaliforniaBalsamic.com, but if you need a substitute, you can use 2 tsp Hickory Flavored Liquid Smoke plus 2-3 Tbsp of your favorite reduced balsamic vinegar.

PEACH BERRY COBBLER

Early one summer I fell into some fresh home-grown peaches. LOTS of them. I ran out of things to make with them, until I developed this recipe. This became breakfast and dessert almost every day until the peach tree was done bearing fruit for the year! It never gets old!

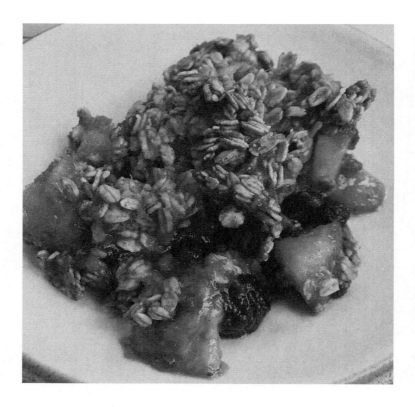

PREP TIME: 12 Minutes

COOK TIME: 25-30 Minutes

YIELD: 4-6 Servings

FILLING INGREDIENTS:

3 cups fresh peaches, sliced

1 cup berries (fresh or frozen, any kind will work!)

1 cup unsweetened applesauce

2 Tbsp ground roasted flax seed *(optional)*

TOPPING INGREDIENTS:

2 large ripe bananas, mashed

1/4 cup almond milk

2 cups rolled oats

1 Tbsp cinnamon

1 tsp cardamom

INSTRUCTIONS:

Preheat oven to 350 degrees.

Combine all filling ingredients directly in a 8×8 or 9×9 baking pan.

In a mixing bowl, combine all topping ingredients.

Put the topping ingredients on top of the filling.

Bake at 350 for 25-30 minutes until topping is starting to brown and fruit is bubbling around the edges.

POWERMINT PATTIES

As with many of my creations, this recipe was inspired by a store-bought product that I had bought a couple times for my daughter, and then instantly regretted it! It was actually the Lara Bar flavor called Mint Chocolate Brownie. It's sweet but not overpowering, and the burst of mint is actually refreshing.

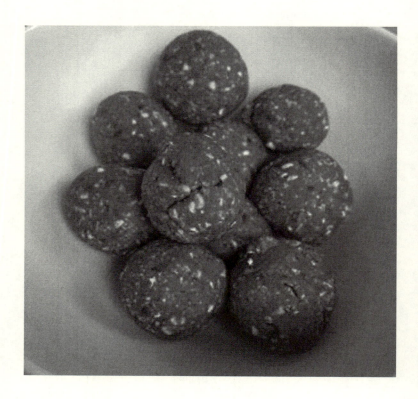

PREP TIME: 10 Minutes

COOK TIME: N/A

YIELD: 2 Dozen Balls

INGREDIENTS:

1 1/2 cups black beans, drained and rinsed, *reserve the liquid

2 cups rolled oats

5 pitted medjool dates (approximately 1/2 cup)

2 Tbsp liquid from the beans

2 Tbsp carob powder

2 drops peppermint oil*

INSTRUCTIONS:

Place all ingredients except the liquid from the beans in a food processor.

Blend 2-3 minutes on low speed, scraping sides occasionally.

Process until mixture becomes crumbly and uniform.

Add liquid from the beans 1 Tbsp at a time until it forms a ball on the blade and is a little sticky.

Form small balls with your hands and flatten if desired to look more like York Peppermint Patties. Store in fridge.

Chef's note: I use Peppermint Essential Oil from Do Terra which is pure, potent, and a little goes a long way! If you're using peppermint flavoring or peppermint oil from another brand, please be sure that it is safe for consumption (to be taken internally), and adjust the quantity as desired. These should leave a nice cool, fresh feeling in your mouth, but not so much that you clear your sinus passages or have your eyes start to water!

STEEL CUT OATMEAL-IN-AN-INSTANT (POT)

Steel cut oats were one of my favorite breakfasts for a long time. But they're so time consuming. It's so easy to walk away from the stove top and come back to a sticky mess. Not anymore! The Instant Pot take the guesswork out of it and you don't have to babysit it.

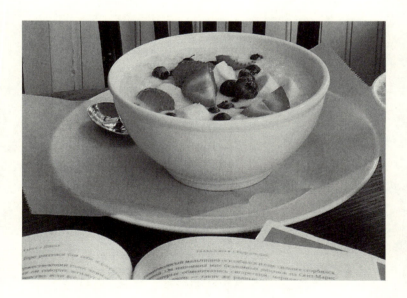

PREP TIME: 3 Minutes

COOK TIME: 25 Minutes

YIELD: 6 Servings

INGREDIENTS:

2 c steel cut oats

1 c unsweetened vanilla almond milk

4 c water

½ Tbsp cinnamon

1 tsp vanilla

½ c dried apples

½ c raisins

INSTRUCTIONS:

Put all ingredients in the Instant Pot.

Cook on manual for 4 minutes. Let pressure release naturally (at least 12 minutes).

It may look too liquidly when you first take the lid off, but give it a good stir and by the time it cools enough to eat, it should be perfect!

VEGGIE LOVER'S PIZZA POTATO

I once was at an Italian restaurant that had nothing but a salad on the menu that would have been compliant. But, they had baked potatoes and pizza toppings. And voila! The Pizza Potato was born.

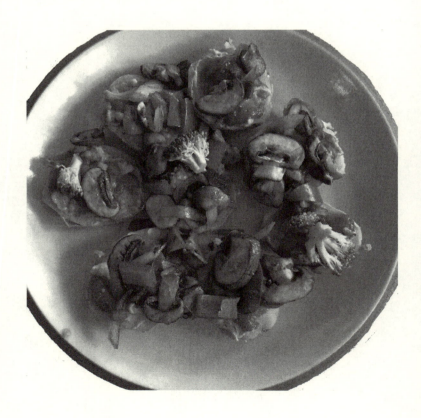

PREP TIME: 10 Minutes

COOK TIME: 50 Minutes

YIELD: 3-4 Servings

INGREDIENTS:

4-6 yukon gold potatoes, baked

2 bell peppers, diced

2 red onions, diced

8 oz mushrooms, sliced

2 c broccoli, chopped

1 tsp onion powder

1 tsp garlic powder

roasted red pepper hummus

2 c marinara sauce

½ c sundried tomatoes

pineapple *(optional)*

crushed red pepper

INSTRUCTIONS:

Preheat oven to 350 degrees.

Bake potatoes 375 degrees for 45-50 minutes.

Chop bell peppers, onions, mushrooms, and broccoli.

Sprinkle with garlic and onion powder, then roast in the same oven 20-25 minutes.

Split open potatoes, smash gently with a fork to form a flat surface.

Spread with hummus and marinara, then top with bell peppers, red onions, mushrooms, broccoli, and sun-dried tomatoes.

For more pizzaz, add pineapple, crushed red pepper, or whatever else you have on hand.

Return to oven for 5 minutes.

ZUCCHINI SAUTÉ

This is a great starter recipe for anyone who is learning to cook without oil. You'll be sautéeing without oil and I think you're going to love it! Master this one and you've got a great staple you can rely on. It's still one of my favorites!

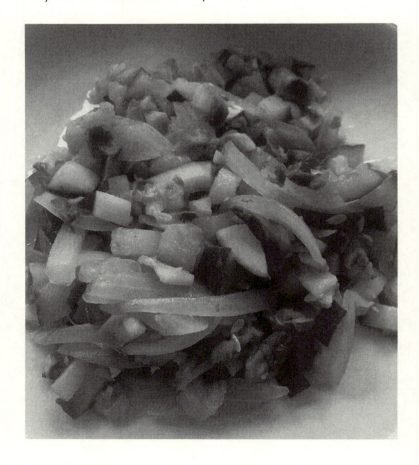

PREP TIME: 7 Minutes

COOK TIME: 10-15 Minutes

YIELD: 2 Servings

INGREDIENTS:

2 onions, diced

3 medium zucchini, diced

8 oz mushrooms, diced

1 tsp garlic powder

1 tsp onion powder

lemon juice or

lemon balsamic vinegar

INSTRUCTIONS:

Cook onions over med-hi heat 2-3 minutes.

Add remaining ingredients and cook another 7-9 minutes to desired tenderness.

Add a squeeze of lemon juice or lemon balsamic vinegar.

Toss and serve.

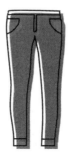

CONCLUSION

The Path Forward

It's in your moments of decision that your destiny is shaped.
~ TONY ROBBINS

Baby Got Back in Her Pants

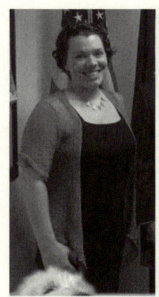
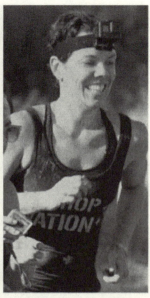
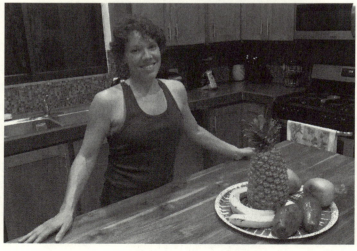

The Path Forward

There are many paths forward, and I urge you to take the one that's paved with proven success. Follow your fellow Voyagers in *TransformU* through the next phase of your journey and begin writing your own success story. Say goodbye to your family history - it is no longer your fate. Say goodbye to endless hours in the kitchen - there is an easier way! Say hello to your new future, where you're in control of how you feel, and how you experience life. You'll be so proud of who you can become, and I'll remind you every step of the way just how amazing you are right this very moment.

THIS, MY FRIEND, IS YOUR MOMENT OF DECISION. WILL YOU JOIN ME?

www.theForeverDiet.org/Transform

About Christin

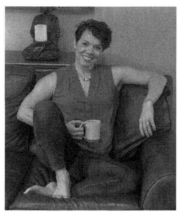

Christin Bummer was diagnosed with hypertension and early insulin resistance at age 32, despite being active and otherwise healthy. It was a massive wake-up call to realize she was walking right down a well-worn path to a family medical history full of heart disease and diabetes. She adopted a whole food plant-based lifestyle, reclaimed her health, lost excess weight, and felt on top of the world! And a few years later she got pregnant and had some difficulties sticking with the plan.

A series of stressful life events pulled her back into old damaging habits, and she found herself really lost, knowing that she wanted to get back on track yet feeling completely unable to do it. Her journey of self-discovery led her to repeatable success, and she's dedicated her life to helping other women overcome similar battles with self-sabotage, insecurities, procrastination, and so much more.

Christin created The Forever Diet online coaching programs now reaching across the globe and she also supports her hometown community with many volunteer endeavors. She is a devoted wife, mom, and dog-mom, and when she's not writing or coaching you'll find her racing up and down the monkey bars with her daughter, hiking in the woods, or daydreaming about their next vacation.

Quick Favor

I'm wondering, did you enjoy this book?

First of all, thank you for reading my book! May I ask a quick favor?

Will you take a moment to leave an honest review for this book on Amazon? Reviews are the BEST way to share these messages of positivity and to encourage others who can benefit from this book as well.